Acute Peripheral Vascular Surgery

Michael Staudacher

With a Foreword
by Professor Ronald J. Stoney, M.D.

With 146 single illustrations
in color (drawings by Wolfgang Rieder)
and 14 black-and-white figures

Springer-Verlag Wien NewYork

Prof. Dr. Michael Staudacher
II. Chirurgische Universitätsklinik, Wien, Austria

Revised and enlarged translation of
„Akute periphere Gefäßchirurgie"
Wien-New York: Springer-Verlag 1983

Softcover reprint of the hardcover 1st edition 1985

Typesetting by Atelier Ing. Dannerer, A-1090 Wien

Library of Congress Cataloging-in-Publication Data. Staudacher, Michael. Acute peripheral vascular surgery. Rev. and enl. translation of: Akute periphere Gefäßchirurgie. 1. Blood-vessels-Surgery. 2. Blood-vessels-Surgery-Instruments. 3. Surgical emergencies. I. Title. [DNLM: 1. Emergencies. 2. Vascular Surgery-instrumentation. 3. Vascular Surgery-methods. WG 170 S798a]. RD598.5.S7613 1985. 617'.413. 85-17328.

ISBN-13:978-3-7091-8804-0 e-ISBN-13:978-3-7091-8802-6
DOI: 10.1007/978-3-7091-8802-6

Dedicated to my beloved wife, Monica

Foreword

During the past three decades, Vascular Surgery has emerged as a specialty within general surgery. Fellowships are now available to equip surgeons with specialized skills for managing various vascular problems. Nevertheless, the vascular surgical emergency, one of the greatest challenges in surgical management, may occur suddenly and at a time and place remote from the highly qualified vascular surgeon or a specialized center where complex vascular treatment is routine. The initial evaluation and treatment must be undertaken by a general surgeon who determines the extent, severity, and urgency of the problem at hand, and hopefully will arrange appropriate transfer to a specialized center if the patient's condition permits.

Urgent problems, on the other hand, demand immediate surgical intervention by the general surgeon if any hope for salvage is to occur. It is in this setting that this volume offered by Professor Staudacher may be of assistance to the general surgeon whose experience in this type of emergency may be limited. This concise, well illustrated volume should serve as a guide to manage the peripheral vascular emergency involving either the arterial or venous system.

The five sections are clearly illustrated and the methodology is described in a stepwise fashion for easy reading. The examples of common vascular emergencies discussed in the final section show the application of principles of exposure, identification of the involved vascular structures, and repair in a clear and concise manner. The successful management of these examples employing basic vascular surgical techniques should serve the reader as a model which can be applied to a specific vascular problem that he faces.

The format makes this an attractive, basic reference for the student, surgical trainee, and surgeon who encounters the occasional vascular emergency.

San Francisco, Calif., July 1985

Ronald J. Stoney, M. D.
Professor of Surgery
Co-Chief, Vascular Surgery
University of California

Preface

Vessels have always instilled an almost mystic awe in physicians. This is in the nature of things, for when large vessels are damaged, it always has serious consequences: the threat of necrosis of parts of the body or a severe blood loss or even bleeding to death. Thus, it is understandable that fellow surgeons who have not had the benefit of basic training in vascular surgery display a certain reluctance towards vascular problems.

Yet, vascular surgery has shown a surge of development since the mid "50"s and today it has at its command a mature basic technique for vascular reconstruction which can be acquired without particular difficulty by any general or accident surgeon - and indeed should be. For if he is unexpectedly confronted with an embolism or some other vascular injury, there is no time to be lost and, if no specialist is available, he must proceed without delay. Such cases are by no means rare. In these cases, he should and could do more than apply a ligature or perform an improvised embolectomy, which will all the more necessitate calling in a specialist, who will then have to repair the damage. None of the participants can be satisfied with this, not the administrator of first aid, not the specialist and certainly not the patient. The best chances of success in acute cases are given only by rapid and correct treatment. Any delay worsens the prospects of recovery.

Nor should we forget situations in which intraoperative iatrogenic vascular injuries occur, for which we must always be prepared. They should not be the cause of panic.

To be equipped for successful vascular reconstruction in such cases, all that is needed is the ABC of vascular surgery and a handful of special instruments.

In this book, the necessary basic knowledge will be described and those instruments will be presented that will put the nonspecialist surgeon in a position to tackle an acute peripheral vascular problem so that he will be able to master it with safety for the patient and to his own satisfaction.

Obviously, not every single one of such cases can be treated in this book. Therefore, we will present the surgical procedures required for the most common and typical diseases and injuries of the peripheral vessels in a readily understandable and easily duplicated manner. Our examples should be taken as models that can be transferred to other situations.

Thus, in this context, it is not appropriate to enter into hemodynamic details, special angiographic techniques, faulty diagnoses, etc. Also, we have refrained from giving detailed references to the scientific literature, which can be found in textbooks of vascular surgery as listed at the end of the book, by those particularly interested.

As to the manner of preparation of the material selected, I believe it is particularly suited to convey the essentials. The course of the operation is captured step by step in drawings, and comments are made in caption form. Each series of pictures is accompanied by the diagnosis of the case in question and a list of postoperative measures.

I have omitted photographs of operations, since these contain too much that is nonessential and thus are not suitable for teaching purposes.

Schematic drawings, such as predominate in many other publications, proved to be oversimplified – easy for those familiar with the field but not clear enough for the inexperienced. I have therefore prepared colored in situ pictures myself, which served as models for the outstandingly successful illustrations of our draftsman, Mr. Wolfgang Rieder.

I hope to have contributed with this book to making reconstruction maximally successful in vascular problems and to making them entrustable to nonspecialists in case of urgency.

I wish to extend my heartfelt thanks to Prof. J. Vollmar of the University of Ulm for his advice and for reading the original manuscript.

My very special thanks are due to my highly honored teacher, Prof. Johann Navrátil, Dr. Sc., who opened up the possibility for me to establish a vascular surgical service in his clinic and to collect the experience which I wish to pass on in this book, and who also wrote the foreword to the first (German) edition.

Finally, the generosity of the management of Eli Lilly International Corporation (Indianapolis, Indiana) must be acknowledged, which made the translation possible.

I also wish to thank the tireless secretaries Mrs. Brigitte Blaschke and Mrs. Waltraud Duminger for all their help and work – work which is all too quickly overlooked once all has been completed.

Last but not least I would like to express my special thanks to Dr. Howard F. Floch for reviewing my manuscript so carefully.

Vienna, July 1985 **M. Staudacher**

Contents

The Vascular Surgical Emergency 1

1 Occulsion 3
Arterial Embolism 3
Arterial Thrombosis 4
Acute Venous Thrombosis 5
Acute Thrombosis of the Axillary Vein 6
The Tourniquet Syndrome 6
2 Aneurysm 8
True Aneurysm 8
False Aneurysm 9
Dissecting Aneurysm 9
3 Trauma 9
Open Vascular Injuries 10
Closed Vascular Injuries 11
Iatrogenic Vascular Injuries 12
4 Compression or Alteration of Vessels Caused by Tumor Formation 13

Minimal Emergency Instrumentarium 15

1 Gelpi's Retractor 18
2 Metzenbaum's Scissors (Modified) 18
3 Potts' Vascular Scissors 18
4 Atraumatic Forceps 20
5 Walton's Atraumatic Needle Holder 20
6 Walton's Atraumatic Needle Holder (Detail) 20
7 Halstead's Clamp 22
8 Freer-Kieny's Dissecting Spatula 22
9 Scalpel (No. 11 Blade) 22
10 Fogarty's Embolectomy Catheter 24
11 DeBakey's Atraumatic Vascular Clamps 26
12 Mock Needle to Prepare the Bypass Vein 26

Preparation for Surgery 29

Basic Vascular Surgical Techniques 33

1 Plastic Closure of a Longitudinal Arteriotomy with a Venous Patch 34

2 Technique of Venous Patch Plastic Surgery 36
3 Basic Measures Before Finishing a Venous Patch Operation (or any Form of Vascular Anastomosis): "Flushing" 40
4 End-to-End Anastomosis of an Artery (Simplest Method) 42
5 Method of Preparation of the Central Great Saphenous Vein of the Right Leg 44
6 Preparation of a Removed Vein for an Oblique End-to-Side Anastomosis 48
7 Oblique End-to-Side Anastomosis Between a Vein and an Artery 50
8 Oblique End-to-Side Anastomosis Between a Teflon Plastic Prosthesis and an Artery 52
9 Preparation of a Plastic Dacron Prosthesis for a Patch 54
10 Various Forms of Anastomoses Between Plastic (Dacron) Prostheses and Arteries 56

Typical Emergency Situations 59

11 Embolic Occlusion of the Right Common Femoral Artery at the Point of Bifurcation 60
12 Simple Puncture Wound of the Right Femoral Artery 68
13 Severe Penetrating Injury of the Common Femoral Artery . . . 70
14 Tearing of the Large Saphenous Vein from the Femoral Vein . 74
15 Severe Penetrating Injury of the Common Femoral Vein 78
16 False Aneurysm of the Common Femoral Artery 84
17 Thrombectomy of the Right Femoral Vein 88
18 Exposure of the Popliteal Artery 94
19 Acute Occlusion of the Popliteal Artery by a Thrombosed True Aneurysm 98
20 False Aneurysm of the Axillary Artery 102
21 Embolic Obstruction of the Cubital Artery 108
22 Open Luxation of the Lower Arm with Tearing Out of the Cubital Artery 114
23 Operation for Inguinal Hernia with Injury to the Right Common Femoral Vein 118
24 Injury of the Axillary Vein During Mastectomy 128
25 Injury of the Common Iliac Vein During Removal of a Female Genital Carcinoma 134
26 Closed Fracture of the Shaft of the Humerus with Injury of the Brachial Artery 142
27 Exposure of the Axillary Artery Distal to the Clavicle for Grafting an Emergency Axillo-femoral Bypass 146

28 Emergency Exposure of Right External Iliac Artery 152
29 Spanning an Infected Vascular Wound in the Right Groin with an Extra-anatomical Iliaco-femoral Bypass 156
30 Injury of the Superficial Femoral/Popliteal Artery with an "Awl" While Boring Through the Thigh Bone 158
31 Injury of the Right Common Carotid Artery in Tracheotomy . . 160

References 165

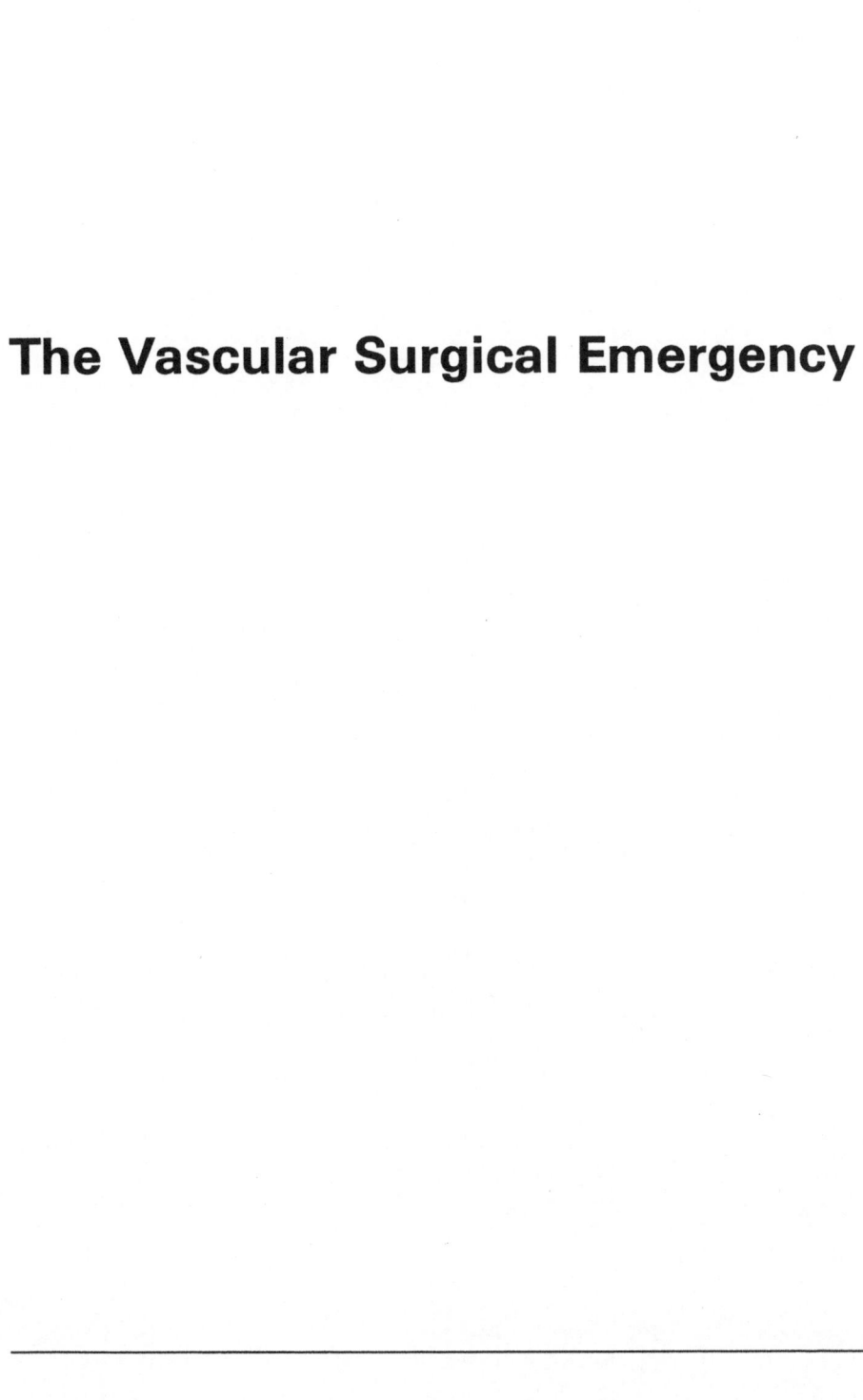

The Vascular Surgical Emergency

First, we will present those possibilities that bring the general surgeon face to face with an emergency situation. In such an emergency, he must decide whether he is ready and in a position to treat a patient with an acute vascular problem himself or whether he has sufficient time to transfer the patient to a specialized service. Aside from purely organizational and time factors, this decision depends upon his surgical abilities.

The following vascular diseases are of interest to us:

- Acute vascular occlusion (from a thrombus or embolus)
- Aneurysm (true, false and dissecting)
- Trauma (open, closed or covered, a distinction being made between opening, penetrating and severing injuries, iatrogenic vascular injuries)
- Effect on the vascular system caused by tumor formation (rare).

1 Occlusion

In this book, we will discuss only acute vascular occlusion, since chronic forms are generally referred primarily to angiologic or vascular surgical services.

In arteries, we distinguish mainly between arterial embolism and arterial thrombosis. In veins, there is only local venous thrombosis produced on the spot.

Arterial Embolism

In typical cases, diagnosis is made on a purely clinical basis and easily. The patient always makes reference to sudden pain towards the extremities, which is very violent and enters deep into the patient's consciousness. The extremity becomes cool and pale, the patient can no longer walk or move his arm. After a time, there are also sensory disturbances and finally disturbances in motility. Pratt's five "P's" may be recalled at this point:

pain
pulselessness
pallor
paresthesia
paralysis

These symptoms, and particularly their sudden appearance, indicate an embolic arterial occlusion. For differential diagnosis, we should also consider phlegmasia cerulea dolens, for, in such cases, there may also be pulselessness with a relatively rapid onset. This will be discussed in greater detail below.

If symptoms of acute embolic arterial occlusion are present, the source of the embolism must be sought. It is often attributable to atrial fibrillation, mitral valve defects, earlier cardiac infarctions or prior vascular diseases:

Accordingly the clinical diagnosis of arterial embolism is generally insufficient, and angiography is advisable in order to be able to

a) rate the influx and
b) exclude arteriosclerotic vascular changes and thus arterial thrombosis.

In cases that leave no doubt angiography can also be dispensed with.

Arterial Thrombosis

Here, we are dealing mainly with thrombosis of the femoral artery, which may occur in this region with signs similar to those of arterial embolism. The diagnosis cannot definitely be made on a clinical basis. Often, we are helped by references to prior intermittent claudication, caused by arteriosclerotic vascular changes, which have now led to a sudden thrombotic occlusion of the vessels. In contrast to arterial embolism, the onset of an arterial thrombosis is not so sudden and brutal, because pre-existing vascular stenoses have already given rise to collateralization of the incipient occlusion. Thus, the symptoms of acute ischemia will be milder.

In cases of arterial thrombosis an effort should be made to obtain angiograms, for often in thrombotic occlusion a thrombectomy alone is not sufficient and the occluded area in which marked vascular changes already exist must be spanned by a bypass operation.

However, it should not be regarded as an error if an arterial thrombosis is operated on without angiography, since by removal of the thrombus, the status quo, with which the patient can live as before, is re-established. Nevertheless in such cases a postoperative anticoagulant treatment must be administered at all costs. Thereafter, the factor that had led to the thrombosis must be eliminated. After a successful thrombectomy performed for an arterial thrombosis, the patient should be transferred to a special clinic where it can be decided whether any further surgical procedure (bypass operation or the like) is necessary.

A special form of arterial thrombosis is acute thrombosis of a popliteal aneurysm. This form of dilating arteriopathy, with special localization in the area of the knee joint, is not as rare as is generally assumed. Therefore, a sudden popliteal occlusion, which is identified as such by angiography, may, during the operation, bring the surprising finding of a popliteal aneurysm. A definite clinical sign of the presence of such an aneurysm is a strong pulse on the contralateral side, which raises the suspicion of a popliteal aneurysm that is not yet thrombosed on this side. In the majority of cases, such popliteal aneurysms are bilateral. Because of the intrinsic problems of popliteal aneurysms, they will be discussed in more detail in a special section of this book.

Acute Venous Thrombosis

Once, again, we will deal with acute thrombosis of the lower extremity. In many cases, it is silent and insidious and, linked to some prior surgical intervention (inguinal hernia, gallbladder, gynecologic operations or the like) it may cause a pulmonary embolism. Here, the only help is derived from familiar prophylactic measures, such as treatment with support hose, mobilization and anticoagulant treatment, to reduce the risks of embolism of the pulmonary artery.

A special form of venous thrombosis of the lower extremities is phlegmasia cerulea dolens, in which all efferent veins of a lower limb are blocked by thrombi. This disease in its later stage may be taken for arterial occlusion, since, owing to the severe edema of the extremity, the peripheral pulses are no longer palpable. However, the onset of this disease is not as acute as that of an arterial embolism. A first sign is a severely swollen leg (twice as thick as the other leg), with a bluish livid discoloration. Pain is not as severe as in arterial occlusion and the patient reports more a strong feeling of tightness.

There is often a pressure pain in the area of the popliteal space and the gastrocnemius musculature and on the inside of the leg along the femoral vein. In thin patients, the femoral vein may be painful to the touch in an inguinal, medial direction from the pulse. The common form of phlegmasia cerulea dolens in itself presents no diagnostic difficulties. However, if there is a suspicion of femoral vein thrombosis, a phlebographic examination should be made to detect the extent of the thrombosis in a cranial direction.

The method of phlebography will not be described in much detail here, other than to say that a pressure bandage is placed around the extremity and the contrast medium is injected into a superficial vein of the instep. If this is not possible, the initial segment of the great saphenous vein at the level of the ankle can be exposed under local anesthesia. What is important is that the contrast medium should be injected into a limb tied off by a compression tube so as to force the contrast medium to flow down through the deep veins of the leg.

Even though surgical treatment of thrombosis of the femoral vein belongs in the hands of those experienced in vascular surgery and, as a rule, can be carried out within a period of one week, which offers the possibility of transferring such a patient to a specialized clinic, it has been dealt with in a chapter in a special part of this book, since in case of phlegmasia cerulea dolens, it may be so acute that the peripheral surgeon will be compelled immediately to obliterate it surgically. Another possibility is thrombolysis with streptokinase or urokinase, but fibrinolytic treatment is not possible in freshly operated patients.

Acute Thrombosis of the Axillary Vein

Acute thrombosis of the axillary vein and subclavial vein forms a separate chapter on venous thromboses. This condition is also known as "Paget-von Schroetter syndrome". As a rule, the disease is not recognized, the symptoms being relatively mild and mainly because it is not thought of. It may also happen that the patient who complains of a general feeling of tightness in the hand and of paresthesia is not carefully examined. There is swelling of the lower arm with distinct prominence of the veins on the dorsal side of the hand. Due to collateralization, the outlines of the veins are distinctly visible over the shoulder and chest muscles. The veins run tortuously over the thorax to the other side. This disease occurs in persons of powerful musculature who feel the symptoms in the hand in question after strenuous physical work of athletic exertion. The clinical diagnosis can only be offered as a suspicion, while the final confirmation should come from the phlebogram. This disease should not be tackled by the general surgeon, since, in the majority of cases, collateralization is sufficient and there are no signs of phlegmasia. This clinical picture is only dealt with for the sake of completeness to recall the possible differential diagnosis of acute arterial venous occlusion.

The Tourniquet Syndrome

Mention must be made of the Tourniquet syndrome in connection with acute arterial occlusion of a limb artery. In this, there is a load on the excreting capacity of the kidneys after reopening an arterial occlusion. Depending on the muscle mass cut off from the blood supply during the time of ischemia, as a result of floating-in of muscle fragments, myoglobin, protein, tissue hormones, potassium ions after reopening the circulation, the entire organism is flooded with these breakdown products which is termed the tourniquet syndrome. Since these breakdown products cannot be adequately excreted by the kidneys, renal function is blocked. Therefore, particularly after a prolonged period of ischemia, particular attention must be paid to renal function and to provide abundant infusions. Thus, the longer a limb has been cut off from the blood supply, the greater is the danger of such a Tourniquet syndrome. In general decompression of the anterior quarter by complete slicing of the strong muscular fascia suffices. Frequently it is necessary, however, to slice the fascia medially and laterally on the extensor side and also on the flexor side ("three compartement fasciotomy") to achieve decompression of the muscles.

2 Aneurysm

True Aneurysm

The true aneurysm of an arterial vessel is a spindle-shaped and sac-like dilatation caused by loss of elasticity of the vessel walls. As a rule, the media, that is the middle layer of the vascular wall, is affected by the disease. The musculature of the vessel is destroyed by degenerative or inflammatory changes (arteriosclerosis, syphilis) or by congenital alterations (Marfan's syndrome). This reduces the elasticity of the vascular wall and the musculature is replaced by connective tissue. The connective tissue, however, is not capable of withstanding arterial blood pressure. This causes dilatation of the vessel. There are sites with a predilection for such degenerative dilating arteriopathies, that is to say, these vascular changes occur especially frequently in certain parts of the body. We should mention, in particular, aneurysm of the subclavian artery after its passage through the scalene gap in the neck or after the costoclavicular narrowing, aneurysm of the infrarenal aorta and aneurysm of the popliteal artery after the adductor canal. The main danger of aneurysmal dilatation of a vessel is from rupturing or peripheral embolization by thrombi from the aneurysmal vascular wall. For this reason, an arterial aneurysm is an absolute indication for an operation.

We do not doubt that the general surgeon may be capable, from a purely technical standpoint of treating a rupturing aneurysm of the infrarenal aorta successfully, especially if he has had a period of training in a vascular surgery service. However, the postoperative danger to a patient who has successfully undergone surgery for a rupturing aortic aneurysm is extremely great. Postoperative care requires considerable use of personnel, technology and space (intensive care unit). It would, therefore, be more appropriate to transfer such a patient to a specialized vascular surgical clinic, for which today the helicopter is the means of transportation of choice.

The same applies to the asymptomatic aneurysm of the infrarenal aorta. These patients can be transferred to a special unit and be successfully treated there. For this reason, we have not included the aortic aneurysm in this account. On the other hand, an appropriate section will be devoted in this book to the aneurysm of the popliteal artery, which occurs repeatedly as a surprice finding.

False Aneurysm

This aneurysm is a so-called pulsating hematoma. A penetrating vascular injury must have occurred beforehand, which was, at first, closed off by blood coagulation factors, but then, due to the slackening of this coagulation plug, leads to bleeding into the periarterial tissue. This bleeding is, at first, contained by a pseudomembrane, after which repeated tears occurs in the pseudomembrane, as a result of which the false aneurysm becomes increasingly larger. With this type of aneurysm, the danger of rupturing is particularly great, but there is no danger of peripheral embolism. The indication to operate is absolute. This is why we have included in this book the false aneurysm of the femoral artery, which may occur either as an accident of daily life or as an iatrogenic injury after puncturing a vessel or in angiography by catheter.

Dissecting Aneurysm

There are essentially two forms that are of practical importance. In one form, dissection occurs immediately behind the aortic valve and the wall layers are pushed apart, which means that the blood flow churns on between the media and the adventitia and two lumina are formed after a time. The danger of rupture is extremely great. The cause of these aneurysm is hypertension and arteriosclerosis with or without trauma. Treatment is impossible for the general country surgeon. He should, therefore, attempt to have such a patient with a suspicion of a dissecting aorta transferred to a specialized clinic which is equipped to perform heart operations with heart-lung machines.

In the other form, dissection may occur in the region of the aortic arch, shortly after the point of origin of the subclavian artery-a so-called "tearing point". The site has a predilection for false aneurysms or dissection after so-called deceleration traumas (fall from a great height, car accidents). Neither the aneurysm produced in this manner, at first encapsulated by the tear in the aortic wall, nor the resulting dissecting aneurysm can be operated on a country hospital. Once again, rapid transportation to a specialized clinic by helicopter is recommended.

3 Trauma

A distinction has been made between open and closed vascular traumas and these again have been divided into opening, penetrating and severing traumas. A special part of this chapter will be devoted to iatrogenic vascular injuries.

Open Vascular Injuries

The main feature of the clinical picture in such cases is shock from hemorrhage or outward hemorrhaging. In patients who are not too old, bleeding from a severed vessel of larger caliber (such as the brachial artery) may already have stopped by the time the patient reaches the surgeon. Ischemic pain is no longer felt because of the blood loss and the protracted state of shock, nor is there any more peripheral ischemic pain. The peripheral pulses are absent and often cannot be palpated on the contralateral side either (which should always be checked!). Here, the most urgent measure is replacement of the circulation. The wound must be precisely excised and rolled up vessel stumps must be sought. After restoration of circulation, the rolled up stump of the central artery can be seen to pulsate in the wound. This and the distal stump of the vessel may be withdrawn far into the tissue due to the elasticity of the vessels. If the pulsating vessel stump is visible, the diagnosis of peripheral, severing arterial injury is certain and an angiogram is, therefore, not necessary.

In open but not severing vascular injuries, there is no such retraction of the vessel stumps. In such cases, hemorrhaging can certainly lead to death from loss of blood. Therefore, the role of the person giving first aid is especially important and he must stop the bleeding by compression with the fingers or application of a compression bandage.

In open venous injuries outward bleeding is again the main feature of the clinical manifestations. If a large vein is severed, the possibility of sealing it up is lost due to contraction of the stump. Venous bleeding may thus be more dangerous than arterial. Even during operations, venous flooding of the area of the operation is considerably more unpleasant than arterial bleeding, which spurts away from the area of the operation. Once again, digital compression is recommended for the person applying first aid, or in the case of injuries to smaller veins, the application of a compression bandage and raising the limb.

How should the surgeon proceed when a patient is admitted with an open vascular wound treated only by digital compression? Here we can only give a few general measures.

- First, the patient should be brought into the operating room.
- Replacement circulation should be administered.
- The blood group should be determined and a transfusion administered.

- Next, the wound should be washed under sterile conditions and the assistants should take over compression of the hemorrhaging vacular wound.
- After a Friedreich's wound excision and a change of gloves, an attempt should be made to expose the vessel above and below the site of the hemorrhage and to clamp it atraumatically (ideal case).

In venous injuries, it is best to block the vein above and below by compression with a sponge stick. Next, an attempt is made to mend the vascular wound with an atraumatic 4/0 or 5/0 continuous suture. If above/below clamping is not successful, the bleeding is taken care of in the open state. The assistant compresses the afferent vessel with a finger and the suture is applied during hemorrhaging, which must be suctioned off with an electrical aspirator. These two methods are always effective, especially when, after the first part of a U-suture, the thread is tightened and held taut so that the second part of the suture can be made with better control of the bleeding.

Closed Vascular Injuries

The closed (covered) vascular injury, which often occurs in association with bone-soft part traumas, may present considerable differential diagnostic difficulties. Perfusion, sensitivity and motor function should be checked without fail in a fracture.

Various types of injuries may be present: impalement of a vessel by a broken bone fragment. In such cases, peripheral perfusion may still persist, but there is a severe vascular injury, threatening the limb. It should be stressed that in fractures of the extremities with a conspicuously growing hematoma, rapid drop of the hematocrit and deterioration of the status of the circulation, an angiogram should be made without fail and quickly.

Diagnostic aids are merely aids. Doppler ultrasound and oscillography are among the best means to determine whether a conjectured arterial injury is still losing blood. If possible, isotope angiography may be extremely helpful in discovering closed vascular lesions. These examinations, however, should always take place in comparsion with the healthy slide. Neither method of examination tells us anything about the quantity of blood that flows through this vascular area. Venous occlusion plethysmography cannot be carried out on an injured limb.

Thus, if there is a suspicion of a covered arterial injury, an angiogram should be made. Angiography today is such a wide-spread procedure that we can refrain from giving a detailed account of it here.

The surgical care of a vascular injury detected by angiography should always be aimed at reconstruction of the injured vascular segment. An anastomosis should by no means be forced. Instead, the vessel stumps should be resected until healthy segments are found, after which reconstruction should take place by implantation of a venous graft (see p. 144).

Iatrogenic Vascular Injuries

Iatrogenic vascular injuries play a special role today. This is due to the fact that in large hospital installations with their modern, invasive diagnostic procedures, they can never be completely ruled out and, therefore, they must be taken into account.

The vascular injuries from angiograms or catheterization are dealt with in this book (stab injuries and false aneurysm of the femoral artery), even though they rarely occur in a general hospital.

Be that as it may, unexpected iatrogenic injuries of larger vessels, which can occur in routine operations, are unpleasant for any surgeon. In such cases, the proper conduct of the surgeon is of paramount importance. There is no universal rule and only general guidelines can be offered. If there is strong hemorrhaging, there is a suspicion of an unintentional injury to a large vessel. The same rules apply as to the open vascular injuries referred to above.

- Finger on the hemorrhaging spot and maintenance of calm.
- Preparation of an electric aspirator.
- Preparation of an atraumatic needle holder with atraumatic 4/0 or 5/0 monofilament suturing material.
- Assistants take over digital compression of the bleeding.
- An attempt is made to expose the injured vessel above and below the site of bleeding and to clamp it atraumatically.
  In venous injuries compression with sponge sticks is safer and less damaging. Sharp, injurious clamps should never be used.

When the above procedure is followed, it is possible, in most cases, to deal with the iatrogenic vascular injury and to re-establish normal blood flow. If this is not possible, the vessel should be tied above and below the site of the injury and the patient should be speedily transferred to a specialized clinic.

In summary, it is stressed, once again, that iatrogenic vascular injuries nowadays should no longer be treated by final ligature of a large vessel, if a limb or an organ is threatened thereby.

4 Compression or Alteration of Vessels Caused by Tumor Formation

This chapter can be kept relatively short, since such cases are seldom severe, acute emergencies and with careful prior examination, compression of a vessel by a tumor is known before the operation. It is mentioned merely for the sake of completeness that especially in the area of the pelvis minor there are tumors that infiltrate the vessels or compress them from outside, thereby causing either venous congestion or inhibition of arterial perfusion. In such cases, however, the possibility is given to transfer the patient to a specialized hospital where with collaboration between the tumor surgeon and the vascular surgeon the appropriate therapy can be undertaken. Should, nevertheless, an injury to a large vessel occur, the same basic rules apply as to iatrogenic vascular injuries.

Minimum Emergency Instrumentarium

Vascular surgery cannot be performed correctly without a certain number and selection of special instruments. If vessels are operated upon with unsuitable instruments, considerable damage may be caused.

The "atraumatic" instruments generally used are 18–22 cm in length. Experience has shown that in vascular operations on the limbs, this length is the most advantageous both for the hand of the surgeon and for manipulation at the site of the operation. In the case of deeper surgical sites-such as the aorta-obviously longer instruments are needed (25–28 cm).

Atraumatic instruments by definition should cause no injury. Nevertheless, considerable damage can be done with them if we proceed roughly with damage to tissues.

These special instruments (mainly forceps and needle holders) have special corrugations on their gripping surfaces (jaws) made of special steel or hard metal, shaped differently from the usual ones. The forceps known as "diamond jaw" have proved especially efficacious.

Operations other than directly on the vessel should not be performed with these atraumatic instruments. For "normal" preparation of the vessels, general surgical instruments should be used, to be replaced by the special instruments only upon opening the artery or manipulations on the vessel itself. If possible, the whole vascular wall should not be held with the forceps, but only the adventitia or the periadventitial tissue. This is extraordinarily important when veins are being operated upon or when veins are being prepared for a patch or bypass and have to be held.

A basic rule to be observed is: the less often a vessel is handled, the better. This is often overlooked due to mistaken zeal on the part of assistants.

In the following, we will describe the instruments that represent an adequate minimum instrumentarium for a surgeon who only wishes to, or must, deal with vascular surgery in isolated cases. In this connection, mention is made of the "Heidelberg vascular surgical emergency instrumentarium", which roughly corresponds to our recommendations, but contains a number of additional instruments beyond the essential basic equipment.

The instruments listed here should always be in readiness in the form of sterile sets in the operating room so as to be immediately available in case of need:

Gelpi's retractor (1 superficial, 1 deep, 20 cm long)
Atraumatic forceps (2, 18 cm)
Walton's atraumatic needle holder (1, 18 cm)
Halstead's clamp (1, 18 cm)
Freer-Kieny's dissecting spatula (1, 18 cm)
Stabbing scalpel, No. 11 blade
Metzenbaum's scissors (modified, 1, 18 cm)
Pott's vascular scissors (1, 18 cm)
DeBakey's atraumatic vascular clamp (2 x 2, 12 and 18 cm)
Fogarty's embolectomy catheters (various sizes)
Mock needle (our own design) or the like (1)
Monofilament suturing material (3/0, 4/0, 5/0, 6/0 with double reinforcement)

1 Gelpi's Retractor

This retractor is especially suitable to keep the edges of the wound open (in some cases, an ordinary retractor can also be used). The pointed ends of the two arms have a pronounced downward curve (ca. 70°) and are bent outward to form hooks.

When retracting, the arms are firmly anchored in the tissue without traumatizing it. This retractor is available in a shallow and deep version and in various lengths. A length of ca. 20 cm and depth of 4 or 8 cm is ideal. It has the added advantage that anastomosis thread cannot become caught up if the retractor lock is covered with a slightly damp cloth during suturing.

2 Metzenbaum's Scissors (Modified)

Metzenbaum's scissors, somewhat modified (ca. 18 cm) are slightly arched and should not be too sharply pointed.

It has special "diamond edge" cutting edges of stainless steel and allows accurate cutting.

These scissors should not be used to cut ligatures or threads.

3 Potts' Vascular Scissors

Potts' angled (60°) scissors (ca. 18 cm) are best suited, for instance, in the ductus choledochus, for cutting vessels open after a longitudinal incision (ca. 5 mm) has previously been made in the vascular wall with a scalpel. This instrument is also excellently suited for cutting venous patches or bypass veins.

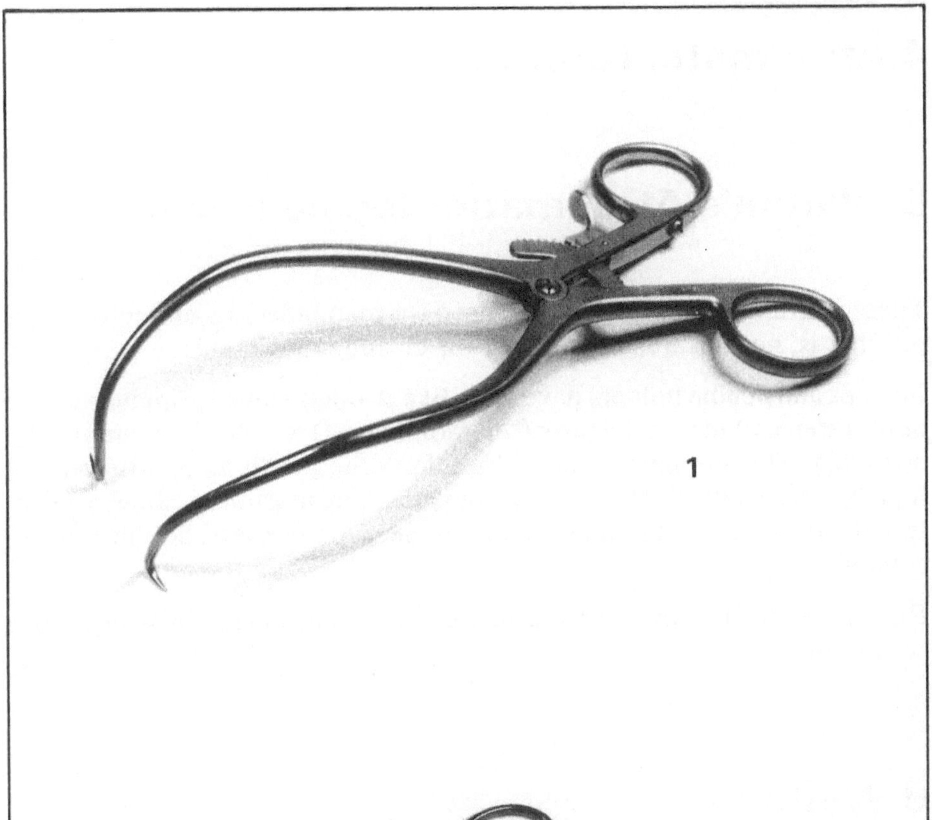
1
2
3

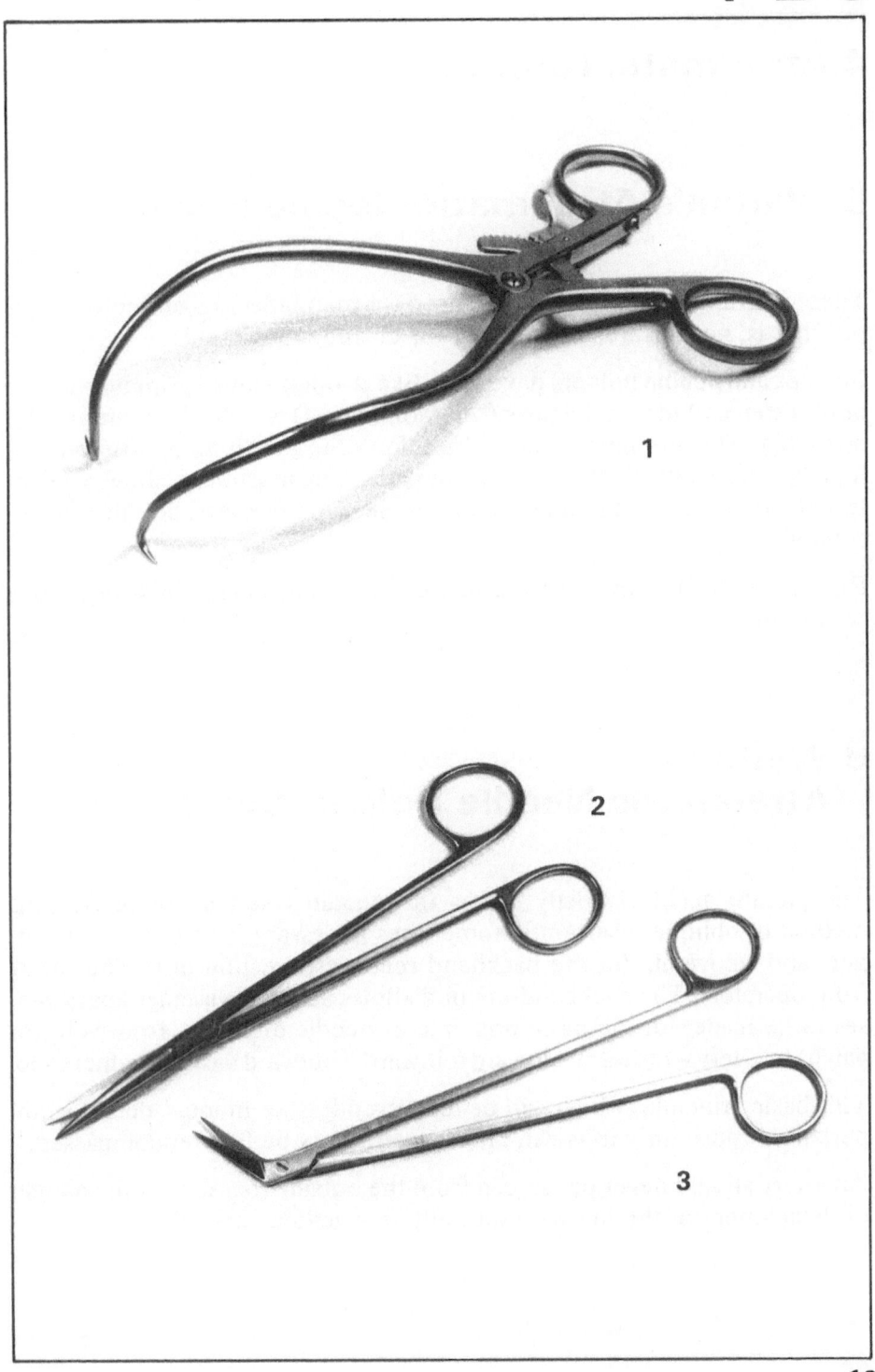

4-5-6

4 Atraumatic Forceps

5 Walton's Atraumatic Needle Holder

These instruments should only be used for manipulations on the vessel itself-that is, not for preparation, nor for closing the wound.

Forceps and needle holders have a file-like strongly ribbed gripping surface of tungsten carbide on the jaws ("diamond jaws") which allows atraumatic operating. This gripping surface also allows the needle to be inserted obliquely. The needle holder has a ratchet lock. The illustration shows a needle with an atraumatic thread (monofilament, 5/0 thickness, double reinforcement).

Recommended length for both instruments: 18 cm, and for deep operations ca. 25 cm.

6 Walton's Atraumatic Needle Holder (Detail)

The picture detail distinctly shows the needle inserted obliquely. This method of oblique insertion is sometimes necessary for anastomosis corners and, above all, for the backhand method (direction of stitches away from operator). The backhand method allows accurate vascular anastomoses to be made, for the basic principle of needle direction, from vein (or patch) to artery - outward - inward - inward - outward - can be adhered to.

This basic principle (which will be discussed further in more detail) is important because only thus can all the wall layers be fully encompassed.

An artery should never be pierced from the outside (because of the danger of detachment of the intima, especially in calcified vessels!).

4-5-6

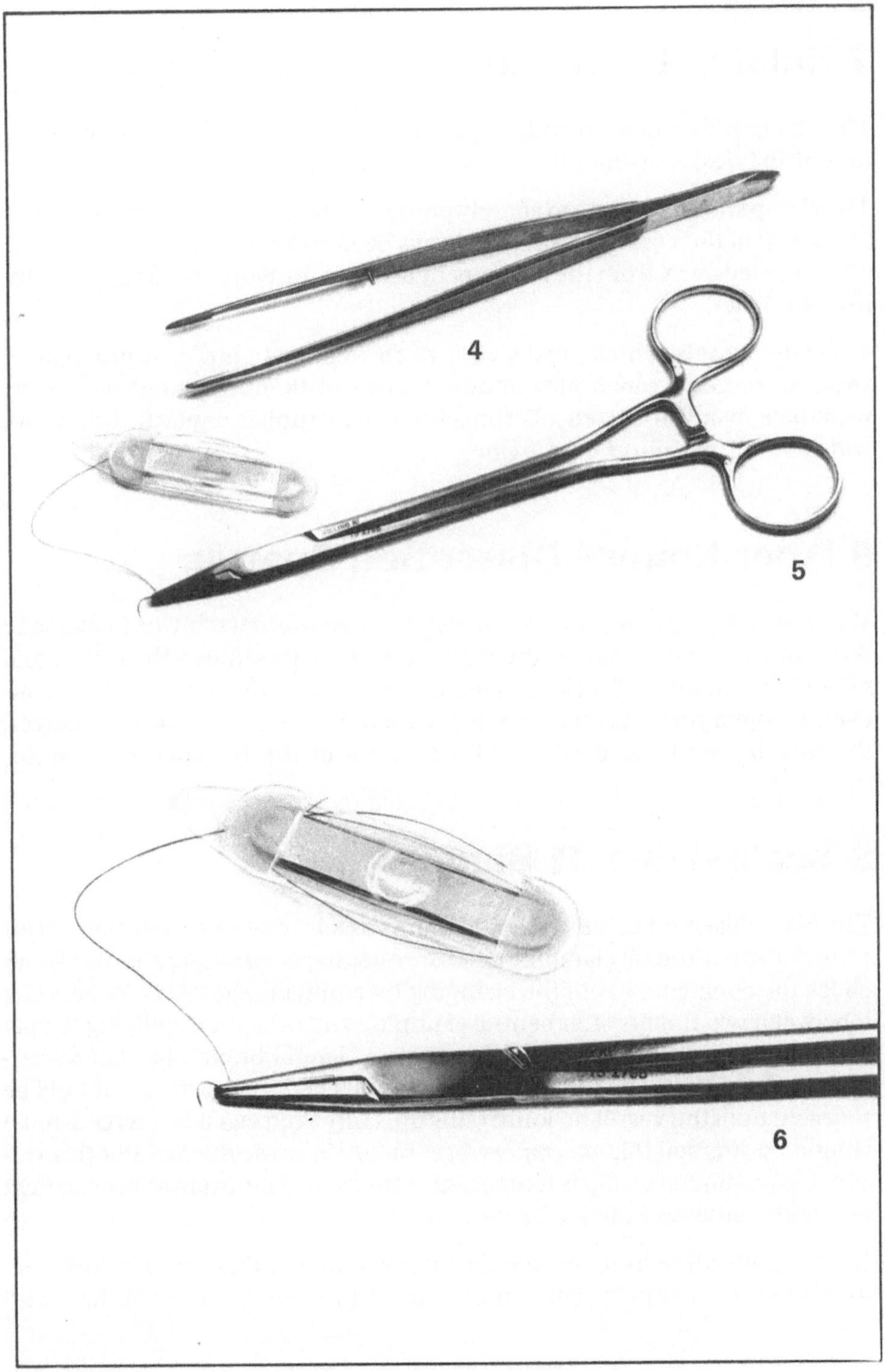

7 Halstead's Clamp

The clamp with a quarter-round arch (ca. 18 cm long), after sharp preparation of the vessels from above, allows them to be tied.

The clamp should not be too sharply pointed, so as to avoid injury to the posterior wall of the vessels. It should always be introduced from the side of the artery turned away from the accompanying vein, to avoid the danger of injuring the latter.

Tying the vessels, which must always be carried out (it is a basic principle of vascular surgery, which also allows control of hemorrhaging) should be with thick, paraffin-coated silk thread or elastic rubber or plastic tubes (not with wick or umbilical cord twine).

8 Freer-Kieny's Dissection Spatula

The dissection spatula (ca. 18 cm long) is used to detach firmly attached thrombi from the intima of the vascular wall or to remove thickened and obliterating masses of intima (open thrombendarteriectomy). Since, however, an open thrombendarteriectomy is an operation not without danger, the spatula should be used only for removal of firmly adhering thrombi.

9 Scalpel (No. 11 Blade)

The No. 11 blade is best suited for opening vessels (obviously only after prior central and peripheral clamping). Before opening a vessel, we should always check the completeness of the clamping by emptying the artery by pressing it between two fingers after central clamping and only then applying the peripheral clamp. If the vessel fills up again, a lateral branch has been overlooked. This should be sought out and tied. The entire procedure should be repeated until the vessel no longer fills up. Only then can it be pierced, but it should be stressed that *an empty vessel should never be pierced.* For this reason, the peripheral clamp is temporarily loosened. The arteriotomy can then be continued with Pott's scissors.

If there is bleeding from the opening of the puncture incision, it is sufficient to compress it manually, suction it off and eliminate the cause of the bleeding.

7-8-9

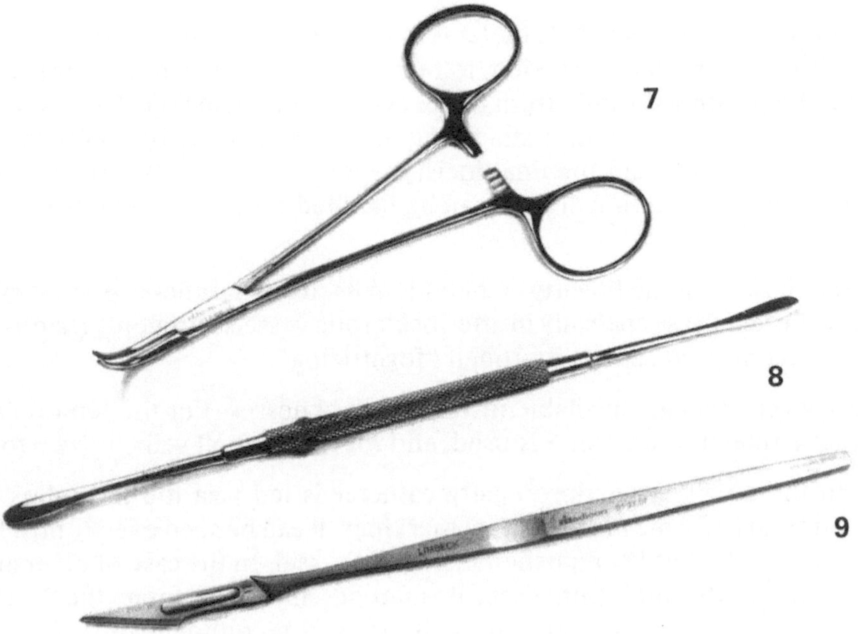

10

Fogarty's Embolectomy Catheter

This catheter has a small rubber sleeve behind the tip which can be expanded by means of an injection syringe attached in the rear, with liquid or air, to form a small spherical ballon.

The purpose of the Fogarty catheter is to be able to enter the vessel far from the site of the embolic occlusion, to remove the embolus, or to extract peripheral separating thrombi from under an embolic occlusion. The classical example is the removal of a straddling embolus of the aortic bifurcation, starting out from small inguinal incisions under local anesthesia. By this means, a life-threatening disease can be handled with a small and harmless intervention.

The application of the Fogarty catheter is in itself not harmless; greatest care should be taken, as especially in arteriosklerotic vessels iatrogenic lesions of the intima may be caused by rough "fogartizing".

Fogarty catheters are available in various thicknesses. For the femoral artery, as a rule, the size 4 or 5 is used, and for the femoral vein, a size 6 to 8.

Ⓐ In the empty state, the Fogarty catheter is led past the thrombus or through it. By means of distinct markings, it can be seen exactly how far the catheter has been pushed inside the vessel. In the case of older and hardened thrombi, sometimes it is not possible to perforate the thrombus with a Fogarty catheter. In such cases, we recommend the use of the older model which is equipped with a thin guide wire, known as a mandrin.

Ⓑ In the full state (preferably filled with air), the balloon catheter is drawn back and removed together with the embolus. Often it is necessary to repeat the Fogarty maneuver several times. It is recommended first to coat the tip of the Fogarty catheter with paraffin before introducing it into the vessel to allow easier sliding of the catheter past the thrombus.

10

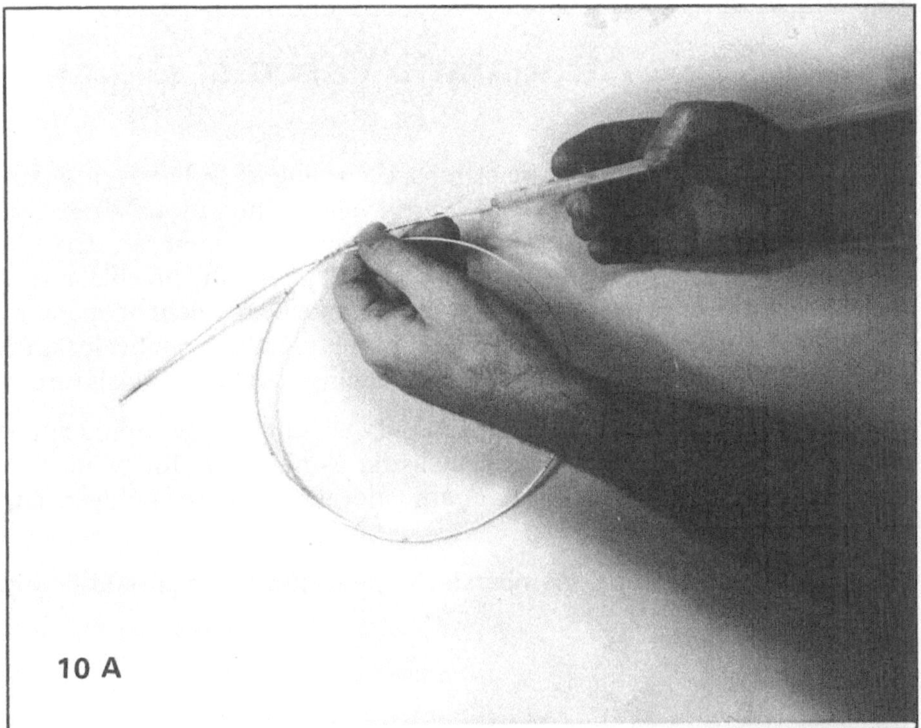

10 A

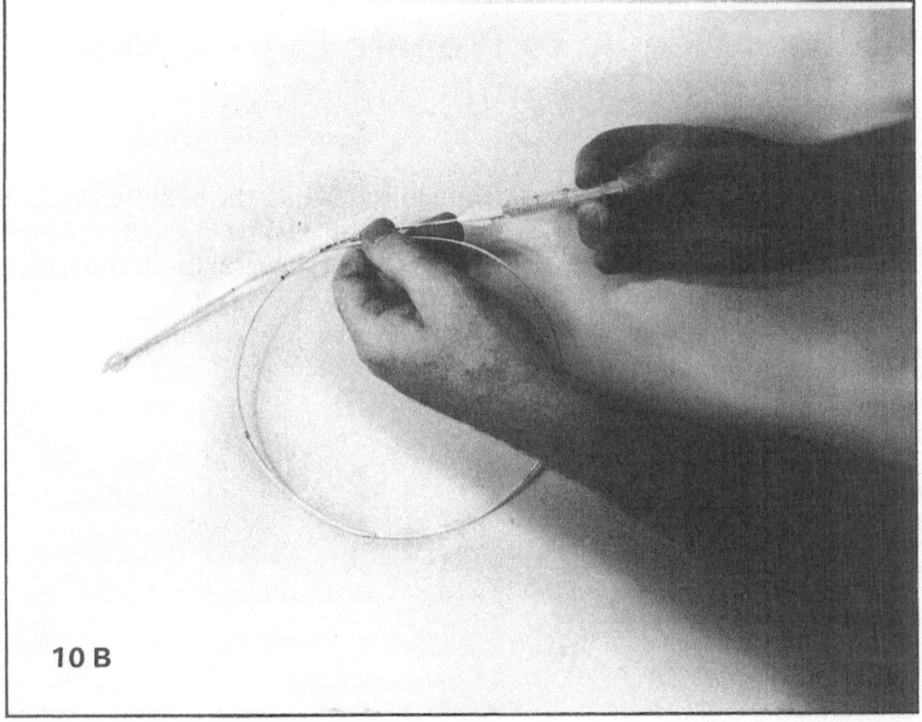

10 B

11 DeBakey's Atraumatic Vascular Clamp

These angled, atraumatic, elastic clamps, according to DeBakey, are standard tools in vascular surgery. They are available in various sizes. The medium size (ca. 18 cm, top) is suitable for the common femoral artery, the smaller size (ca. 12 cm, bottom) for the popliteal artery, the brachial artery, the deep femoral artery. The ratchet locks are outside the field of operation and do not obstruct. Before making a vascular suture, these ratchet locks are covered with a slightly damp cloth to avoid catching the anastomosis thread.

The clamps should not be closed up to the last setting - they should not be allowed to "rattle through" - but only as far as necessary for hemostasis (stage-by-stage clamping). These atraumatic clamps have a ridged jaw, which prevents slippage.

Clamping can be tried on the operator's small finger and should be just slightly painful.

12 Mock Needle to Prepare Bypass Vein (Our own Design)

This canula with a Luer-Look attachment is tied into the peripheral end of the removed vein. It can then be tested for tightness and be slightly dilated. A diluted heparin sulution is used for this (5000 U heparin for 100 ml Ringer solution) (see also p. 46).

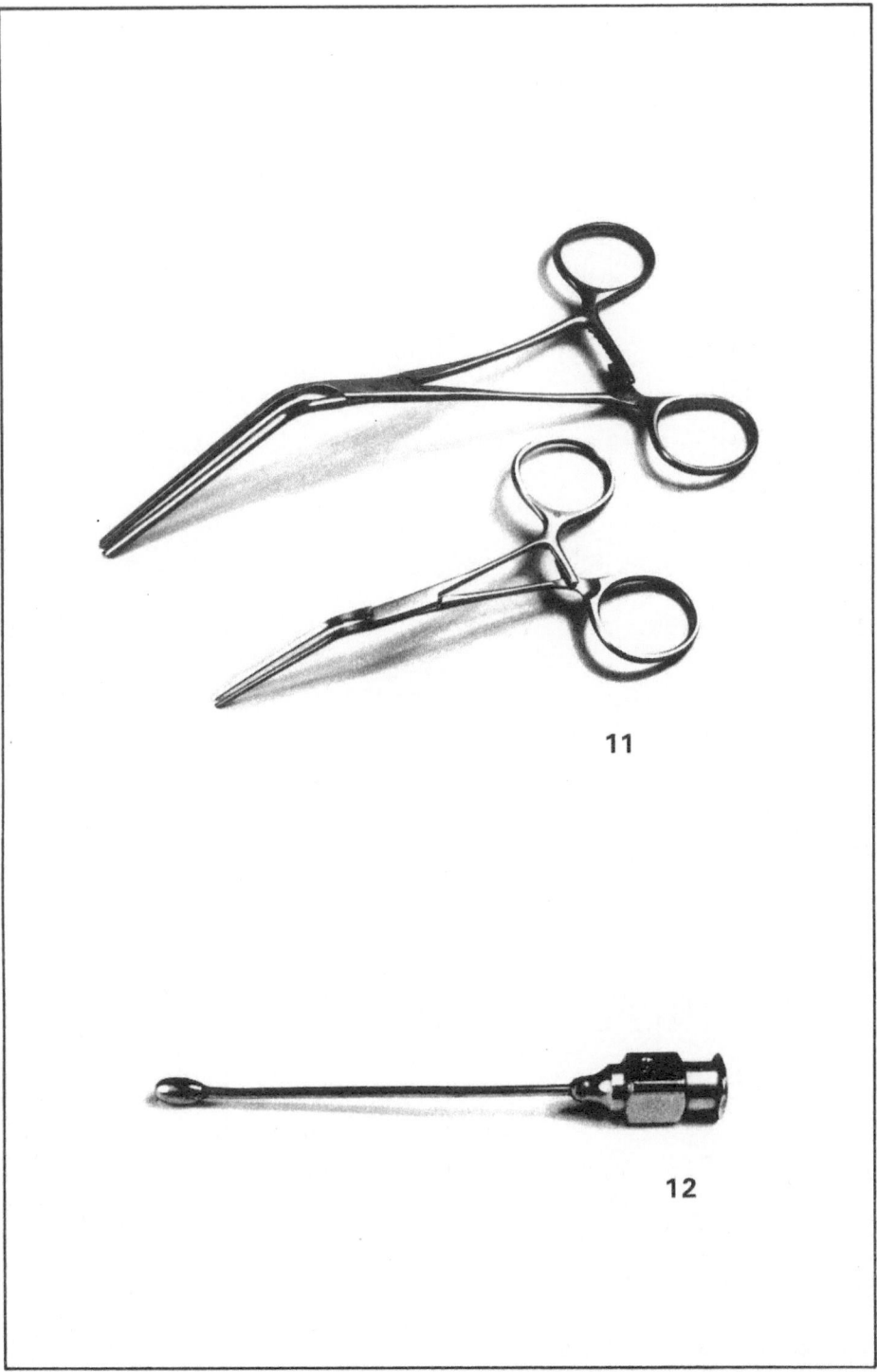

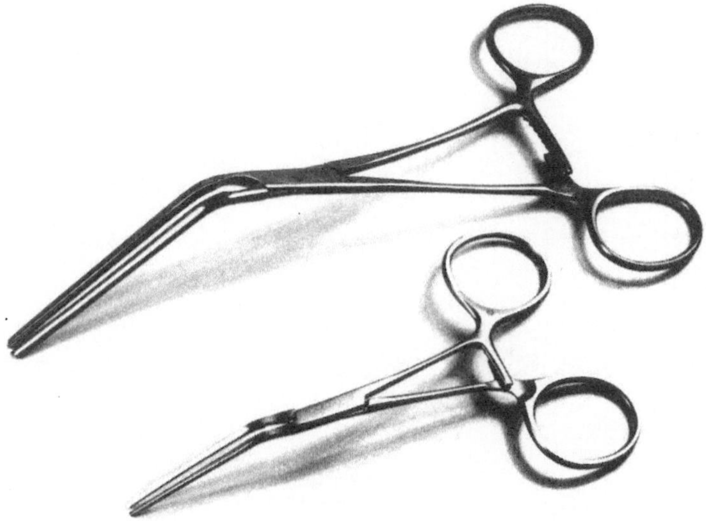

11

12

Preparation for Surgery

Patients with acute arterial occlusion should be administered at least 5000 units of heparin i. v. very soon after admittance to the hospital to keep the danger of renewed embolism or growth of a thrombus (appositional thrombus) low.

It is a basic principle that must be stressed, that in reconstructing a vascular segment the distal and proximal area must also be washed and covered to keep them sterile. In relation to the inguinal region, this means that in addition to the groin, the lower abdomen and the entire limb must be washed until sterile and only the anterior portion of the foot is wrapped in compresses. In this manner, all vascular areas of a limb can be reached and the need for possible later uncovering and redisinfecting of the skin in areas not yet washed is obviated. This may be necessary especially for removal of a peripheral venous patch. In taking care of peripheral vascular injuries it is advisable to prepare also the uninjured leg so as to ensure sterile conditions if pieces of veins must be used to substitute vessels. Commercial preparations can be used as skin disinfectants. Since, in general, in vascular operations there is no covering around the edges of the wound, the skin should be washed at least 6 times as a precaution.

When positioning the patient, he should be placed in a dorsal position. In operations on the upper limbs, such as exposure of the cubital artery, an arm splint or arm support can also be used.

The decision whether to operate under general or local anesthesia depends upon the patient's overall condition and the possibilities of the anesthesiology unit. It is, however, of considerable advantage to use local anesthesia in older patients with defective circulation and cardiac insufficiency, where it should be given definite preference over general anesthesia.

The local anesthesia recommended is a 1 or 2 % procain solution in commercial form without added epinephrine. For adequate suppression of pain, for instance in preparing an inguinal artery, up to 40 ml procain solution may be required.

After local anesthesia or general anesthesia, the vessel is prepared. We should always strive for the most direct route. Sharp preparation is required to keep bruising of tissues and injury to lymph pathways to a minimum (important particularly in the inguinal region).

After exposure of the vessels and before atraumatic clamping, 5000 U heparin is administered intravenously (we omit local heparin blockade before the atraumatic clamp which was formerly used).

This single heparin administration is sufficient in the overwhelming majority of cases. After termination of the operation, the heparin is not neutralized, that is to say, we do not administer protamine chloride or protamine sulfate. In most cases, the administration of heparin is continued postoperatively, 3–4 times 5000 U depot-heparin for 3–4 days. The main resaon is, however, prophylaxis of embolism of the pulmonary arteries. In the case histories given as examples, we will discuss the necessary anticoagulation.

In addition the circulation should be adequately supported by infusion of Ringer solution, or, in cases with severe blood loss, by administration of additional citrated blood. Above all renewed infusion of liquid into the patient seems important to avoid coagulation of the blood.

In vascular operations, a brief peri-operative antibiotic prophylaxis is recommended. An appropriate cephalosporin preparation can be used for this in a dosage of 2 x 2 g per day for 3 days, the first dose being administered at the beginning of anesthesia. In our clinic, for some years, we have successfully used Mandol®/Cefamandole (formerly Kefzol®/Cefazoline) and have had virtually no cases of infection. The rate of infection was less than 0.5%.

Basic Vascular Surgical Techniques

1

Plastic Closure of a Longitudinal Arteriotomy with a Venous Patch

Longitudinal opening and transverse stitching (as for instance, the intestine) is not possible in the case of vessels. Therefore, when closing an arteriotomy, it is best to use a graft from a strip of vein (venous patch), which should be taken from the periphery of the trunk of the great saphenous vein. This patch plastic operation should prevent stenosing the artery by the suture. The central great saphenous vein should be left intact because of the possibility of a later need for a vascular operation. Therefore, before a planned vascular operation, the entire leg should be washed until sterile so as to allow us to remove such a vein fragment quickly in case of need. If this is not possible, a piece of an arm vein (cepahlic vein or basilic vein) can be removed for a patch.

We should always strive to close with a patch, since only by this method can we avoid stenosis of a directly sutured artery. This applies most particularly to vessels damaged by arteriosclerosis. In special cases, a plastic patch may also be used, although the venous patch, particularly because of the ideal (identical) inner layer, its good tolerance and low incidence of infection is certainly to be given preference.

Ⓐ Longitudinal arteriotomy of an artery of medium caliber. The edges of the incision are kept apart by means of holding threads to ensure that all wall layers are definitely included by the needle. The holding threads, as well as the suture material, are of monofilament plastic thread (in other words, not braided). They are removed only after fastening the anastomosis thread.

Ⓑ A patch is cut from a peripheral vein. For this, it is best to use Potts' scissors and atraumatic forceps.

Ⓒ A double-reinforced thread is threaded through the patch and arterial wall in the two "corners" (technique: patch-artery, out - in - in - out).

Ⓓ Beginning of continuous suture, in this case, with 5/0 monofilament thread (distance between stitches 2–3 mm). This suturing material makes it possible to loosen the suture during stitching to make sure that all wall layers have been included.

Ⓔ When the patch plastic operation is ended, the thread is fastened in the left corner. We can also sew 3/4 of the circumference with one end of the thread and fasten it at the site of an earlier holding thread.

1

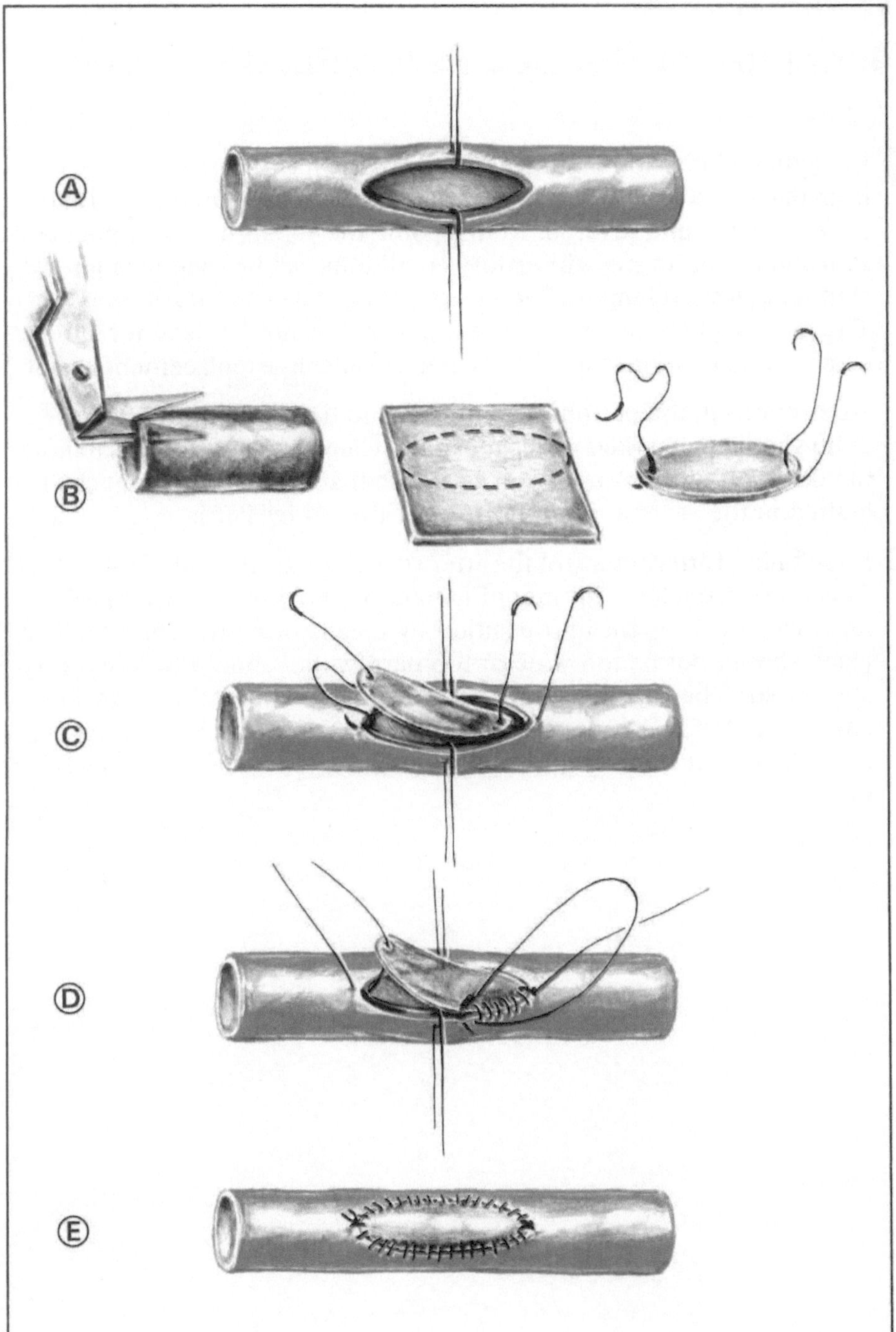

2

Technique of Venous Patch Plastic Surgery

Ⓐ Longitudinal incision on the distal end of the leg. In a medial direction from the inside ankle, the great saphenous vein is sought out, tied at the peripheral end and severed. At this point, the vein is directly under the skin and under normal circulatory conditions can be seen through the skin. The desired lenght of vein is removed. The central stump is tied. The great saphenous vein of the thigh should not be used for simple patch operations, since it might be needed later as a replacement vessel.

After removal, the peripheral end (close to the ankle) of the vein segment should be marked with a mosquito clamp or a suture so as to note the direction of the venous valves and so that the vein segment can be grafted in the reverse position (turned around by 180°).

Ⓑ Longitudinal arteriotomy of the artery (in this case, the right femoral bifurcation), retracted with monofilament plastic thread. The exised venous patch is brought into position by means of corner threads. The patch should not be too wide or too narrow, but should be sewn very slightly stretched so that it does not bulfe forward and later form an aneurysm. A visually, not particularly pleasing-looking venous patch is still better then stenosis after direct suturing of a longitudinal arteriotomy.

Ⓐ

Ⓑ

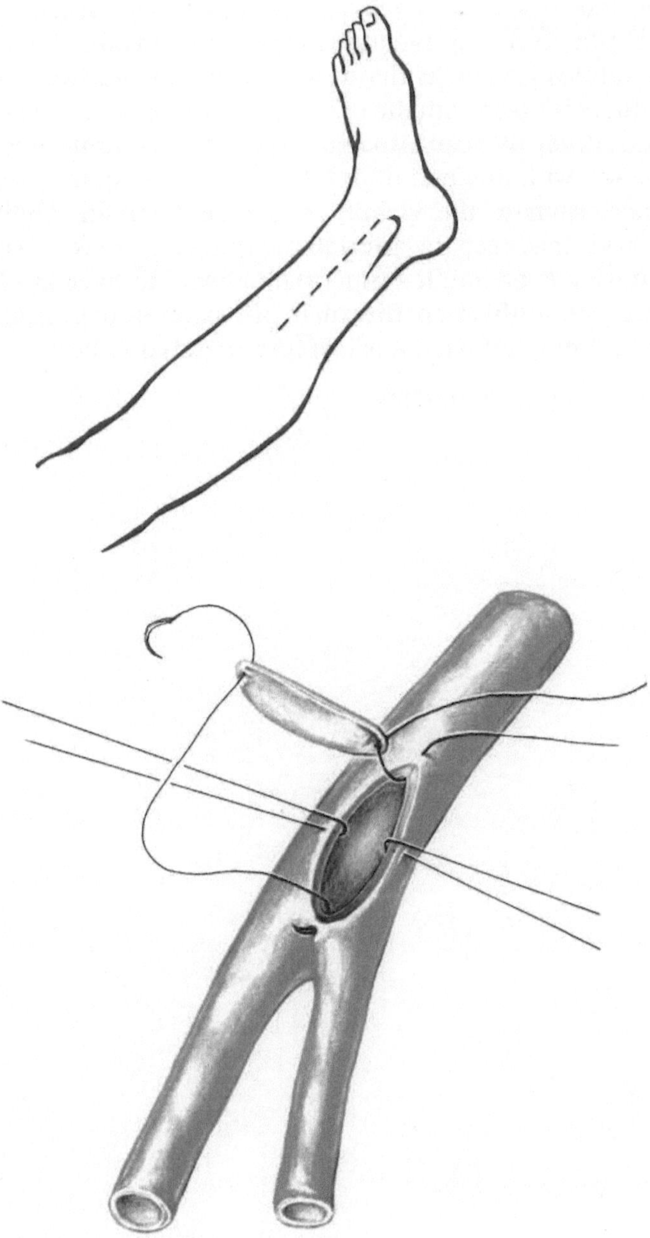

Ⓒ The arteriotomy is retracted with holding threads. A corner thread is fastened (the other serves as a holding thread, and as soon as it is reached by the continuous suture, it is cut off and pulled out) and the first row of sutures is made with one end of the thread. Next, the second row of sutures is made with the other end of the thread and fastened in the second corner. We can also make 3/4 of the circumference of the patch operation with one end of the thread and one quarter with the other and thus fasten in the vicinity of a lateral holding thread. The holding threads that keep the arteriotomy retracted are removed after the entire suturing is ended. It is important always to have available doublereinforced monofilament thread. In our example of a plastic patch operation on a femoral vessel, a 5/0 suture material is best.

Ⓓ The patch is completed.

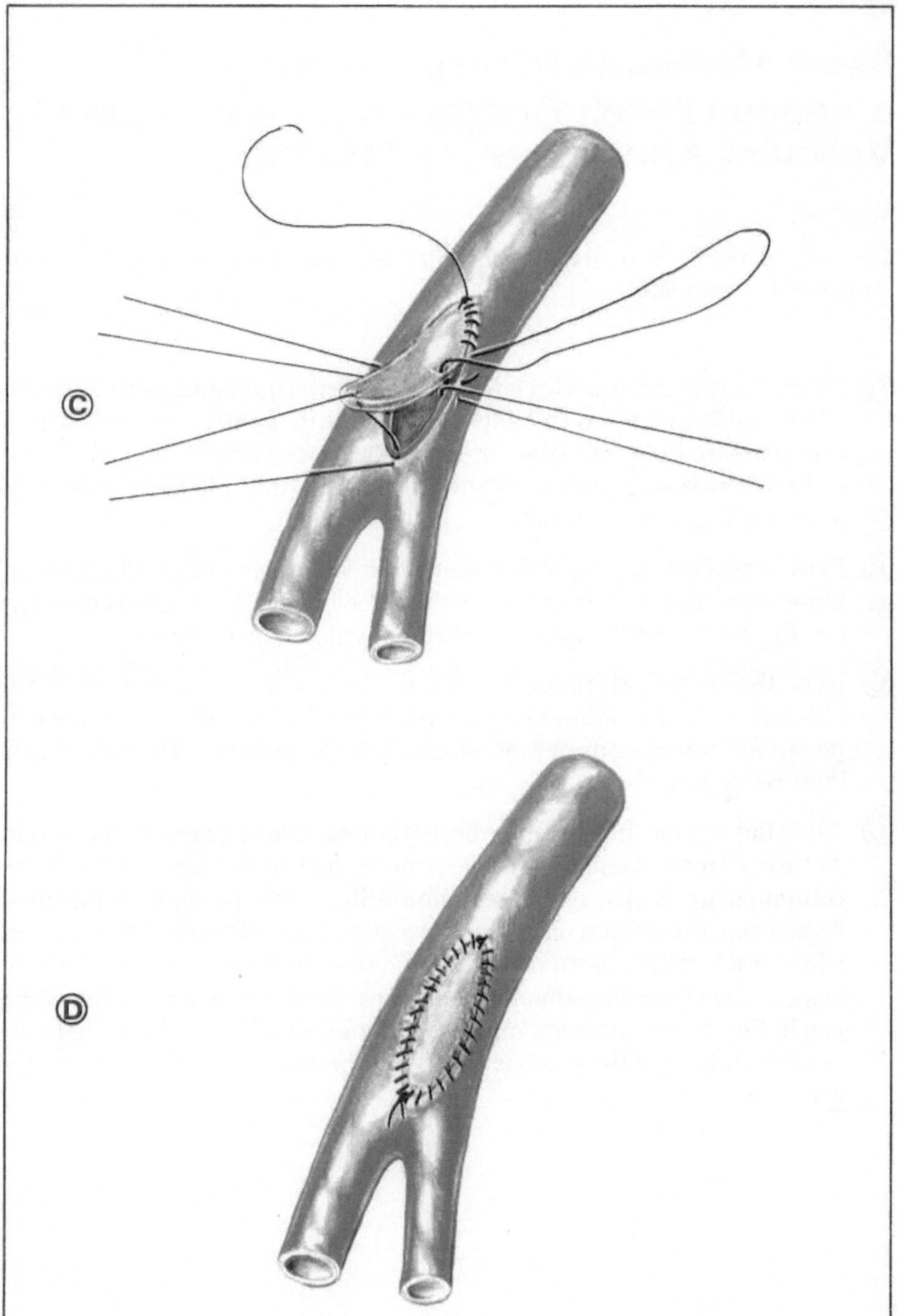

3

Basic Measures Before Finishing a Venous Patch Operation (or any Form of Vascular Anastomosis): "Flushing"

This procedure serves to remove possible local thrombi above and below the clamps and to ventilate.

Ⓐ Artery held by atraumatic clamps. Patch plastic operation with monofilament suture material is ended. The patch is lightly retracted with a clamp before final fastening, the threads are kept loose. This gives rise to a gap between the patch and the arterial wall (this only works with monofilament suture material).

Ⓑ Peripheral clamp is opened (right hand side in picture - direction of blood flow from left to right). The reverse blood flow is allowed to persist for 2-3 seconds, after which the clamp is closed again.

Ⓒ Next, the central clamp is opened (left in the picture). Now the efferent blood flow (which should be synchronous with the pulse) is allowed to persist for 2-3 seconds before the clamp is closed again. The threads are then tightened.

Ⓓ After tightening the threads, the peripheral clamp (right hand side in picture) is opened and only then is the thread finally fastened. Next, the central clamp is also removed. Should there still be marked bleeding from a gap, the central clamp is replaced and the bleeding taken care of with a single stitch. Fastening of a patch sewn with monofilament thread to an empty vessel (atraumatically clamped) can lead to narrowing of the patch. Five to six knots are made. Bleeding from the puncture channels as a rule dries up if the patch is lightly compressed for 2-3 minutes with a dry swab.

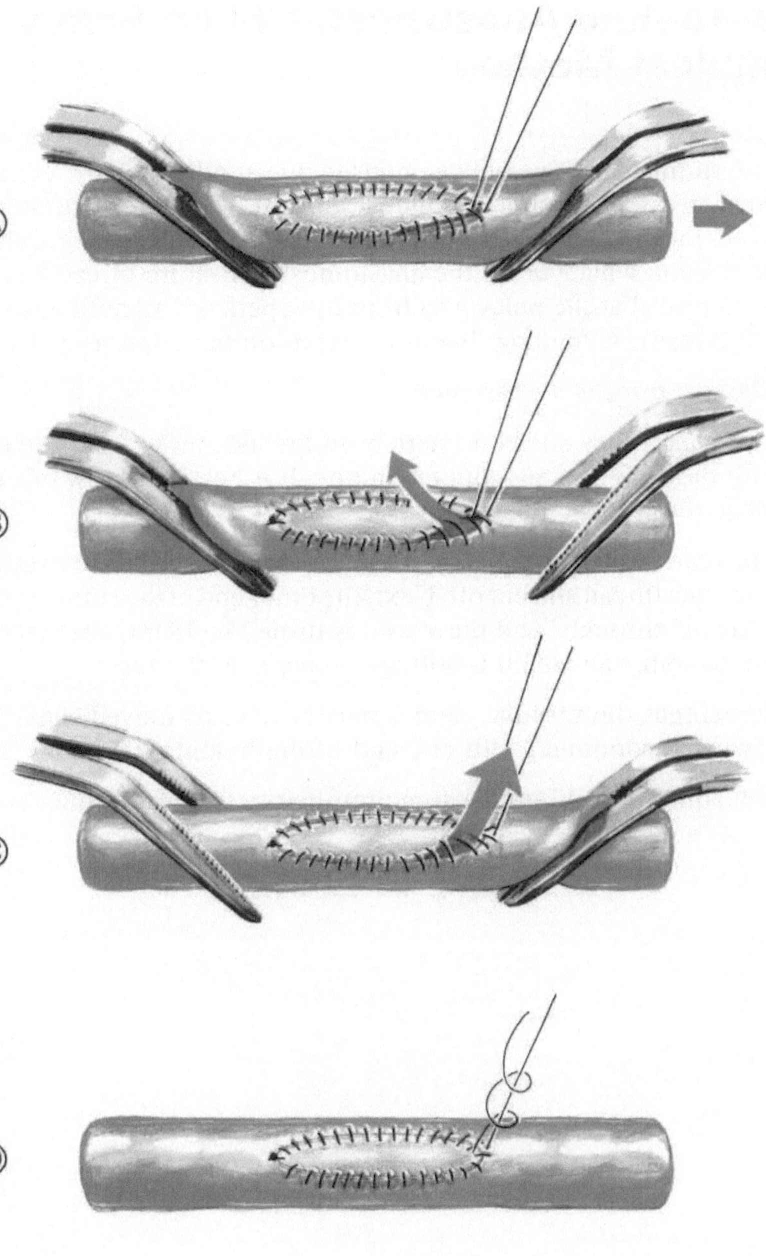

4

End–to–End Anastomosis of an Artery (Simplest Method)

Ⓐ The stumps of the vessel lie opposite one another and the edges of the incision can be straight or oblique (as in B). The oblique anastomosis is easier to perform, since there is less danger of stenosis. There should be no tension whatever on the anastomosis. A sature thread has already been placed at the pole away from the operator (monofilament plastic 5/0 thread). A holding thread is placed on the opposite pole.

Ⓑ The two threads are fastened.

The continuous suture is started on the side away from the operator with the out - in - in - out technique. It is best if the row of sutures is made towards the operator.

Ⓒ The upper wall is completed, the suture thread is fastened to one end of a holding thread and cut off. Next, the other end of the suturing thread is "stitched through" and the vessel is turned by 180° C. In this manner, the bottom wall which is still open comes to the top.

Ⓓ Sometimes the vascular clamps may have to be moved slightly. Next, sewing is continued with one end of the holding thread.

"Flushing" should not be forgotten before final fastening.

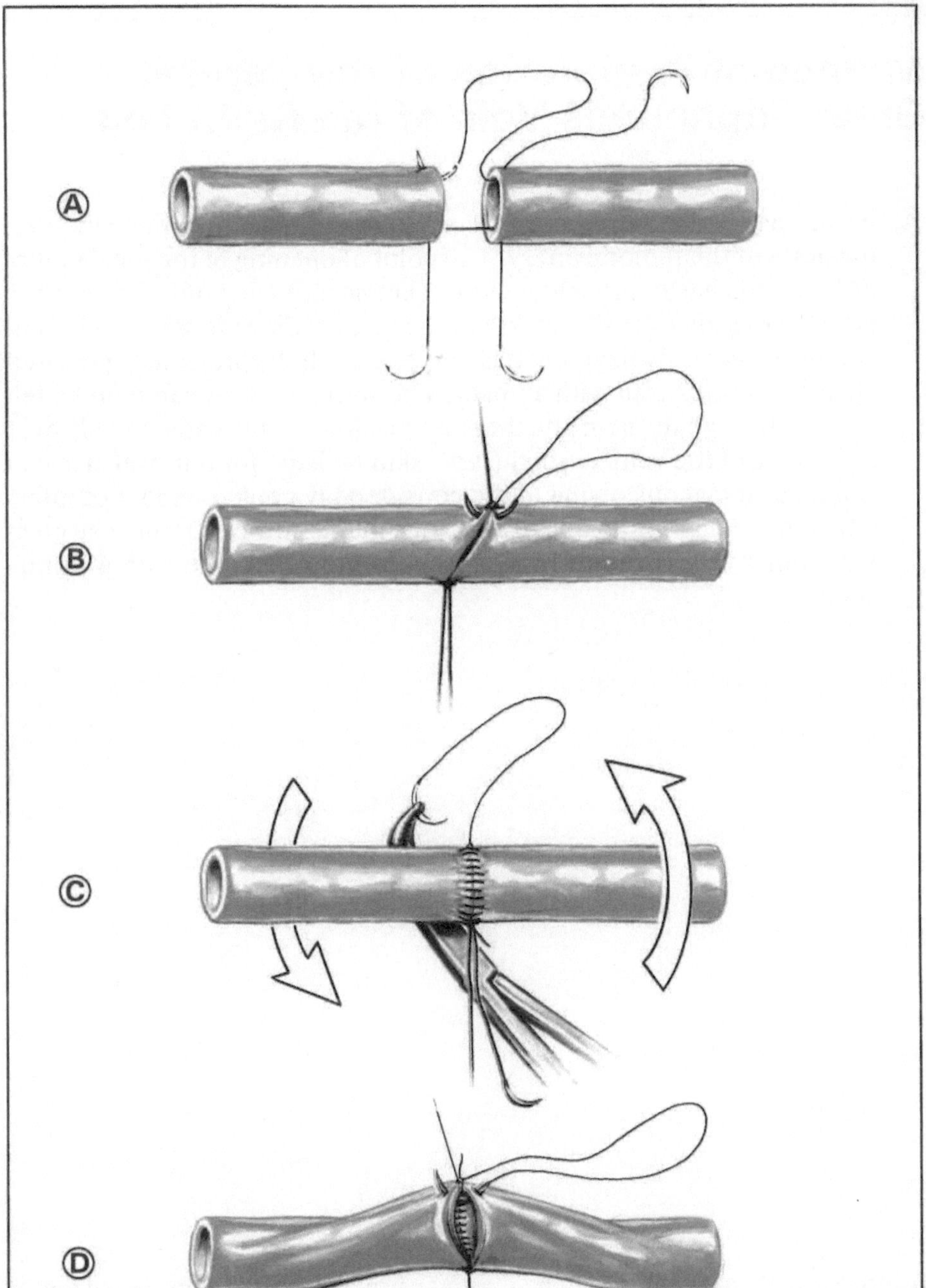
A
B
C
D

5

Method of Preparation of the Central Great Saphenous Vein of the Right Leg

Ⓐ A comma-shaped skin incision is made in the groin just medially from the pulse of the femoral artery. The point of opening of the great saphenous vein is easily prepared. Other skin segments should lie as far as possible exactly over the course of the vein. If they are far from it, skin necroses can easily develop. It is best to stretch the previously prepared great saphenous vein with a finger. The stretched vein can then be felt distally through the skin and the skin incision can be made directly over the course of the vein. A single large skin incision for removal of a vein is not advantageous owing to the considerably greater danger of infection and the possibility of a disturbance in the flow of lymph. The great saphenous vein is removed from the groin to the knee with 4–5 incisions.

Important: Preparation should be as gentle as possible. The vein should not be grasped with instruments. Lateral branches somewhat removed from the main truck (ca. 5 mm) should be tied and cut to avoid constricting rings of adventitia. It is recommended to wind the vein during preparation with a soft rubber sling and keep it in this manner.

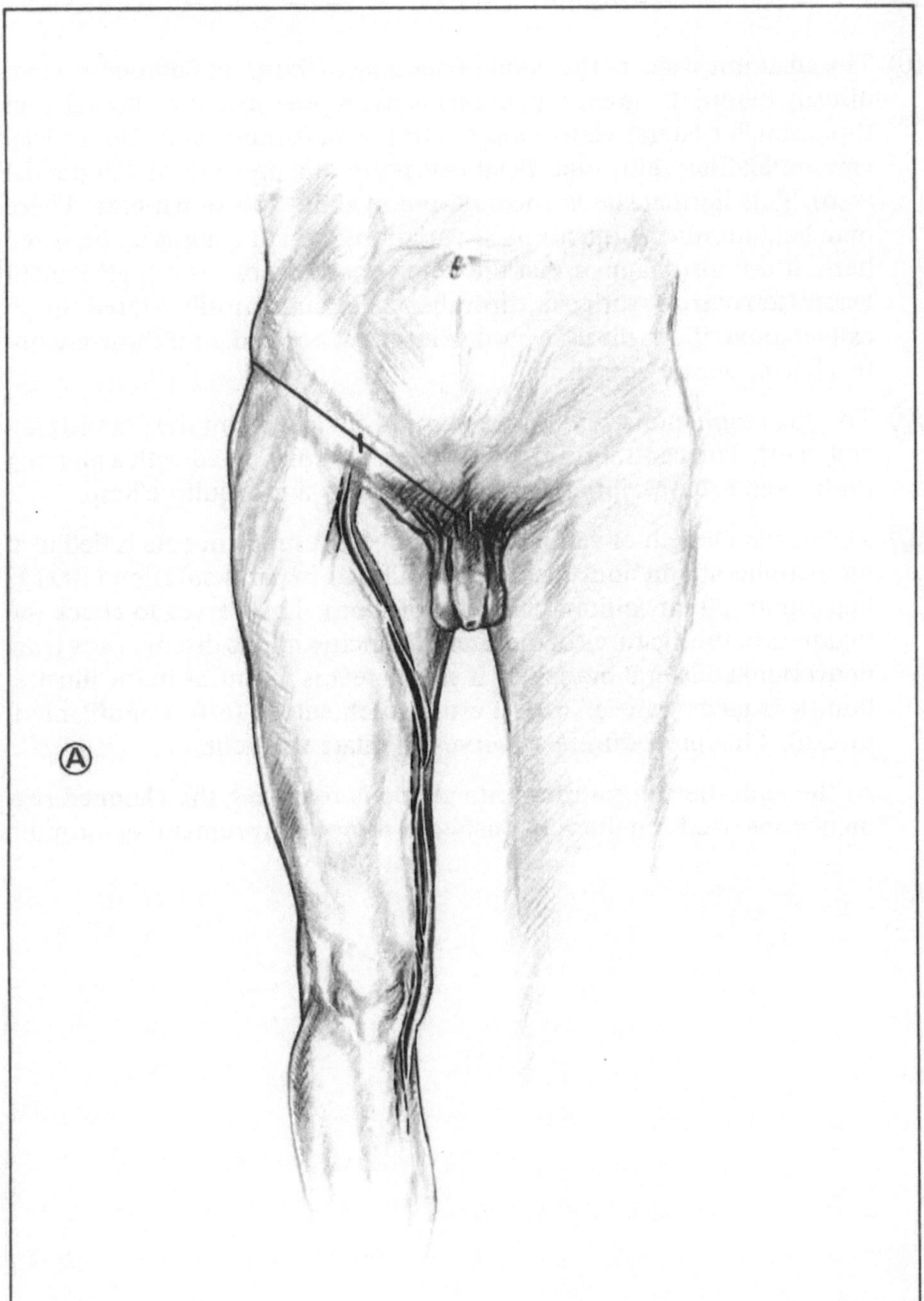

Ⓑ The anatomical site of the point of opening of the great saphenous vein: directly before the great saphenous vein empties into the femoral vein three smaller lateral veins empty into the saphenous vein (superficial circumflex iliac vein, superficial epigastric vein and external pudendal vein). This normal site is encountered in about 70% of patients. There may be a number of anatomical variations, which cannot all be listed here. It can also happen that the vein is not suitable as a replacement vessel (too narrow, varicose, thrombosed, inflammatorily altered, surgically removed). In this case, arm veins must be used, or if these are unreachable, plastic vessels.

Ⓒ The great saphenous vein is clamped and cut just below the entering lateral veins. The central stump of the vein is strongly tied with a piercing ligature and the peripheral stump is held by a mosquito clamp.

Ⓓ The needed length of vein is then removed. A mock needle is tied in at the peripheral end and washed with diluted heparin solution (5000 U heparin to 100 ml sodium chloride solution). This serves to check the tightness of the ligatures of the lateral branches and to discover any tears in overlooked lateral branches. If such a tear is found, as in the illustration, it is taken care of with a cross-stitch suture (6/0 monofilament thread). This procedure also serves to dilate the vein.

At the end, the central mosquito clamp is removed, the clamped segment is resected and the vein washed to remove any remaining thrombi.

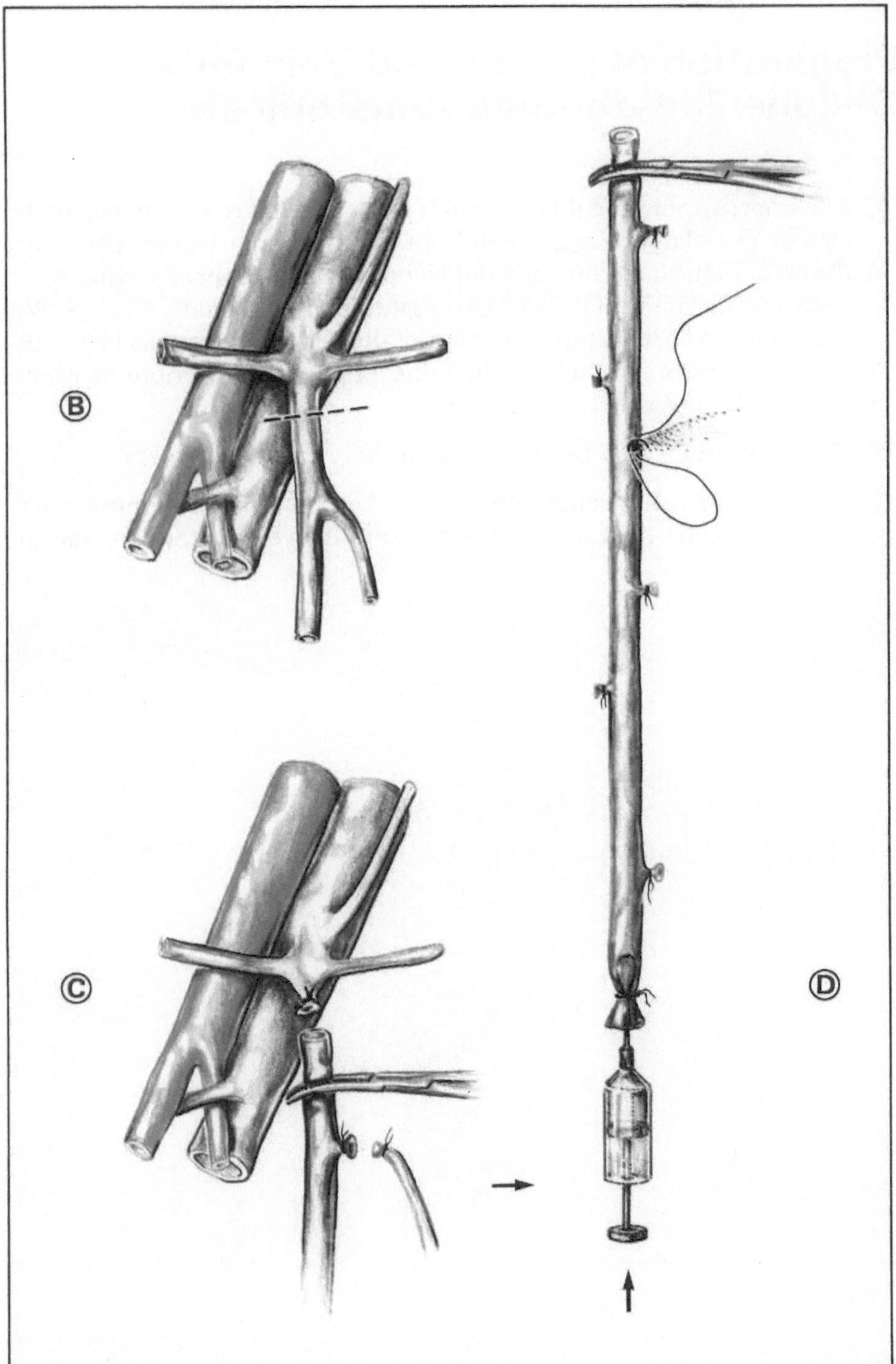
B
C
D

6

Preparation of a Removed Vein for an Oblique End–to–Side Anastomosis

Ⓐ The impermeable and dilated vein is first severed just next to mosquito clamp. The clamped area should not in any circumstances remain on the graft. In the long run, this could jeopardize the proper functioning of such a graft. The vein is then cut longitudinally with Pott's scissors. We should make sure that the direction of the venous valves has been noted. The incision should be of the same length as the arteriotomy which it is supplying (usually 1.5–2 cm).

Ⓑ The corners, created by cutting open the vein, are cut away.

Ⓒ The "corners" of the anastomosis are taken up with 5/0 monofilament threads (double-reinforced) (in - out) and the vein is ready for anastomosis.

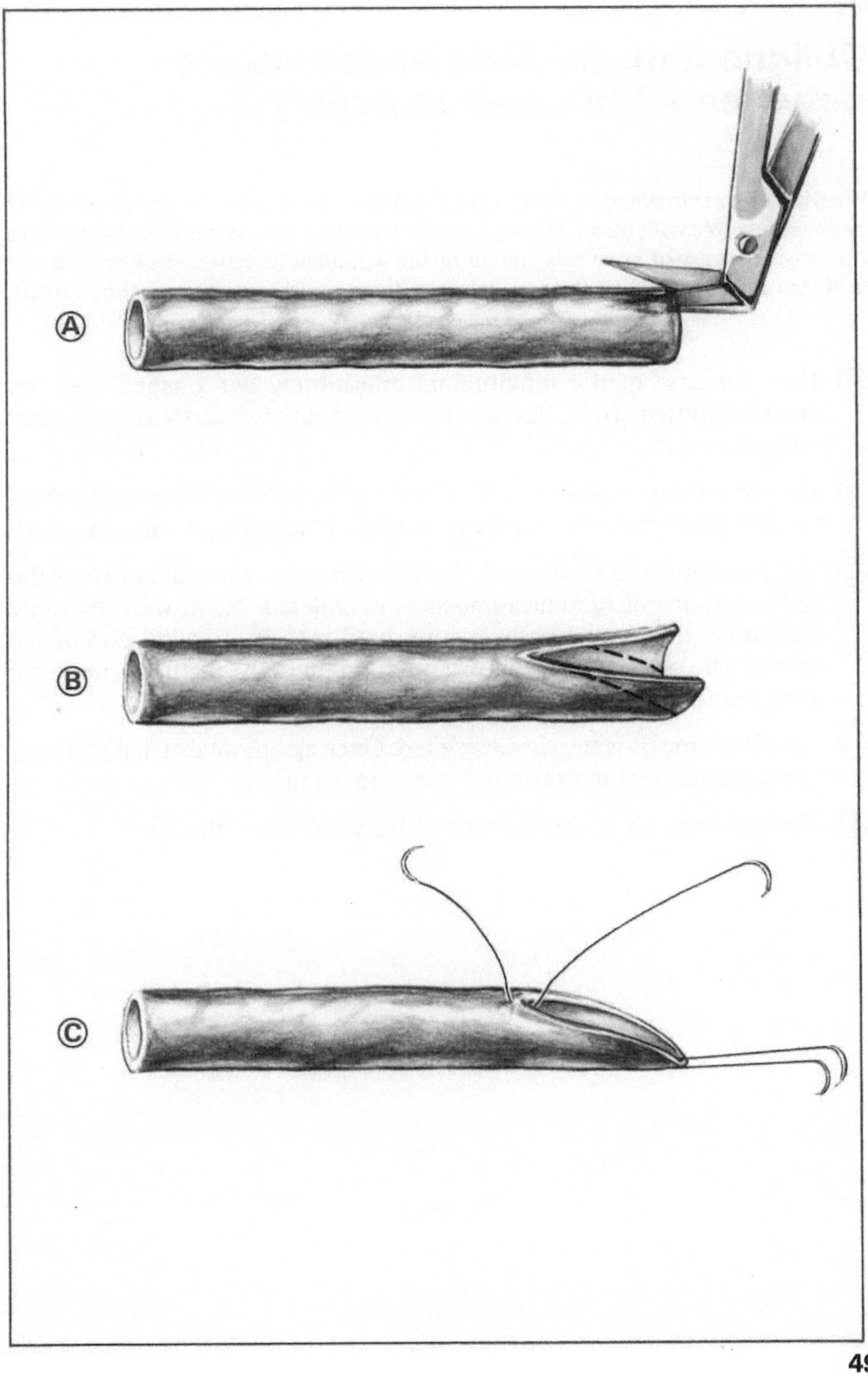

7

Oblique End–to–Side Anastomosis Between a Vein and an Artery

We will not enter in detail into this form of oblique anastomosis in typical emergency situations. We will, nevertheless, present it, for in a case of unavoidable ligature of a vessel because of a severely contaminated wound or infection, the limb in question can only be saved by a bypass operation (from healthy vessel to healthy vessel).

Ⓐ The "corners" of the longitudinal arteriotomy are grasped with the thread as shown in 6 C. The arteriotomy is kept retracted with two lateral holding threads.

Ⓑ The anastomosis is started with a continuous suture (5/0 monofilament thread) in a direction of stitches from vein to artery (out - in - in - out).

Ⓒ The anastomosis is continued. With the first end of the thread 3/4 of the circumference of the anastomosis is completed. Next, with the same technique, the anastomosis is continued with the second end of the thread. The corner thread shown on the right in the picture is removed once the row of sutures reaches it.

Ⓓ The anastomosis is nearly completed. Once again, we can distinctly see the technique (vein-artery, out - in - in - out).

Ⓔ The anastomosis is completed and fastened after "flushing".

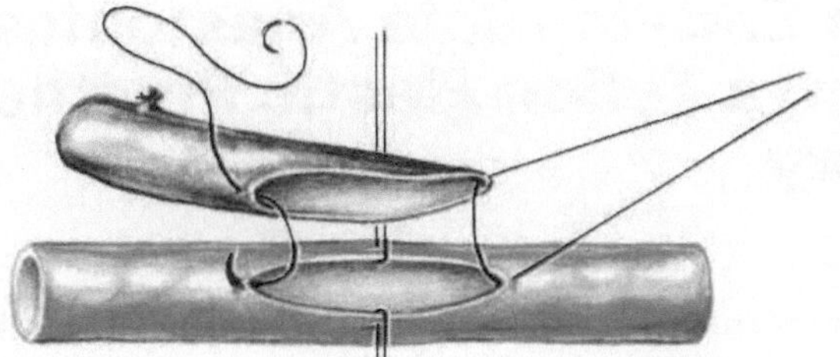

Ⓐ

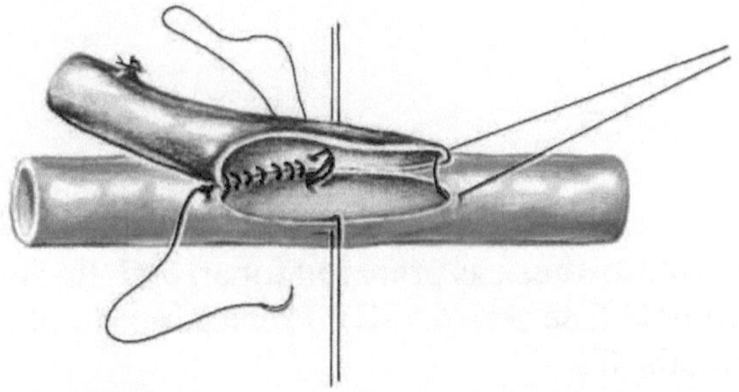

Ⓑ

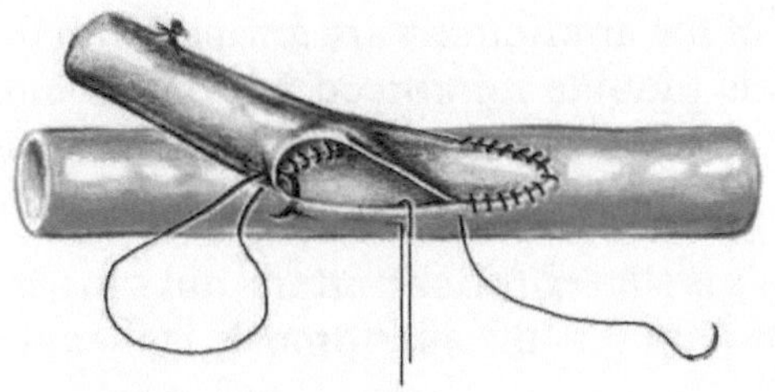

Ⓒ

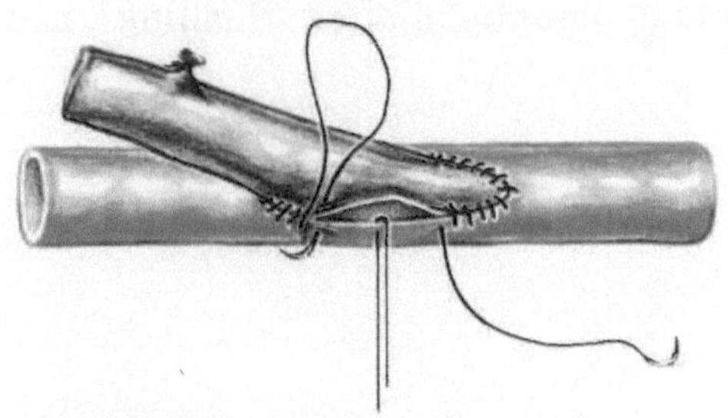

Ⓓ

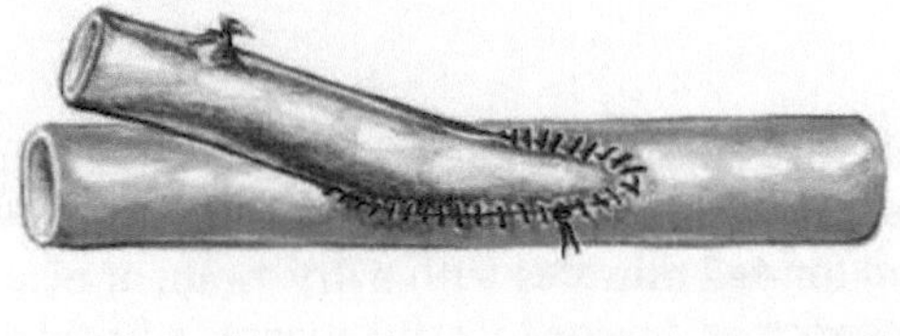

Ⓔ

8

Oblique End–to–Side Anastomosis Between a Teflon Plastic Prosthesis and an Artery

Plastic prostheses (of Teflon or Dacron) should basically not be used for contaminated or infected wounds. This form of anastomoses is presented here to allow saving of a limb in case of a closed vascular injury or in the absence of a suitable vein.

Ⓐ The vascular prosthesis is prepared for an end–to–side anastomosis and cut accordingly (see also 6A–C). Preclotting is not required for such a Teflon prosthesis.

Ⓑ The "corners" of the arteriotomy are grasped with the "corner threads" of the prosthesis (double reinforced 5/0 or 6/0 monofilament thread should be used). The arteriotomy is retracted with lateral holding threads.

Ⓒ The anastomosis is started (plastic-artery, out - in - in - out). The principle of the technique for this anastomosis is identical to 7A–E.

Ⓓ The anastomosis is completed after "flushing", as in 7E.

Important: The puncture channels of Teflon prostheses bleed longer than, for instance, the puncture channels of a veno-arterial anastomosis. The anastomosis should be compressed for 4–5 minutes with a dry swab, or else, fibrin sponges may be used. If bleeding cannot be stopped by this means, a fibrin adhesive strip always has the desired effect.

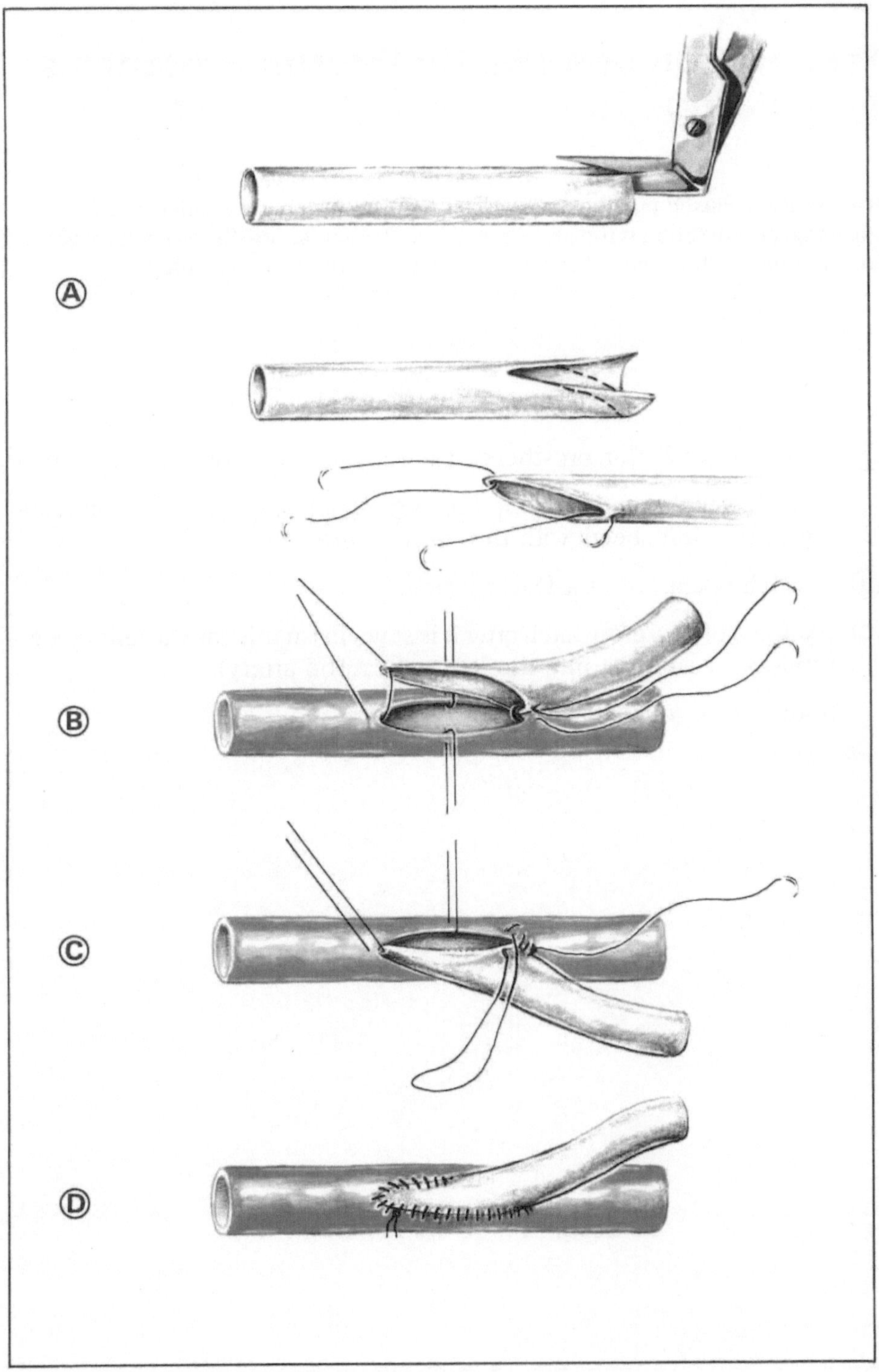

9

Preparation of a Plastic Dacron Prosthesis for a Patch

Important: Plastic prostheses must not be used for open vascular injuries since the danger of infection is too great. An infected vascular prosthesis leads inevitably to softening of the edges of the anastomosis and to severe bleeding.

Ⓐ In contrast to Teflon prostheses, Dacron prostheses must be preclotted.

The exact technique of preclotting is generally given in the accompanying instruction sheets with the vascular prostheses.

Ⓑ A patch is cut out of a Dacron tube.

Ⓒ Example of a Dacron patch after it is sewn in (in this case, a common carotid artery running into the internal carotid artery).

Suture technique as in 1A–E.

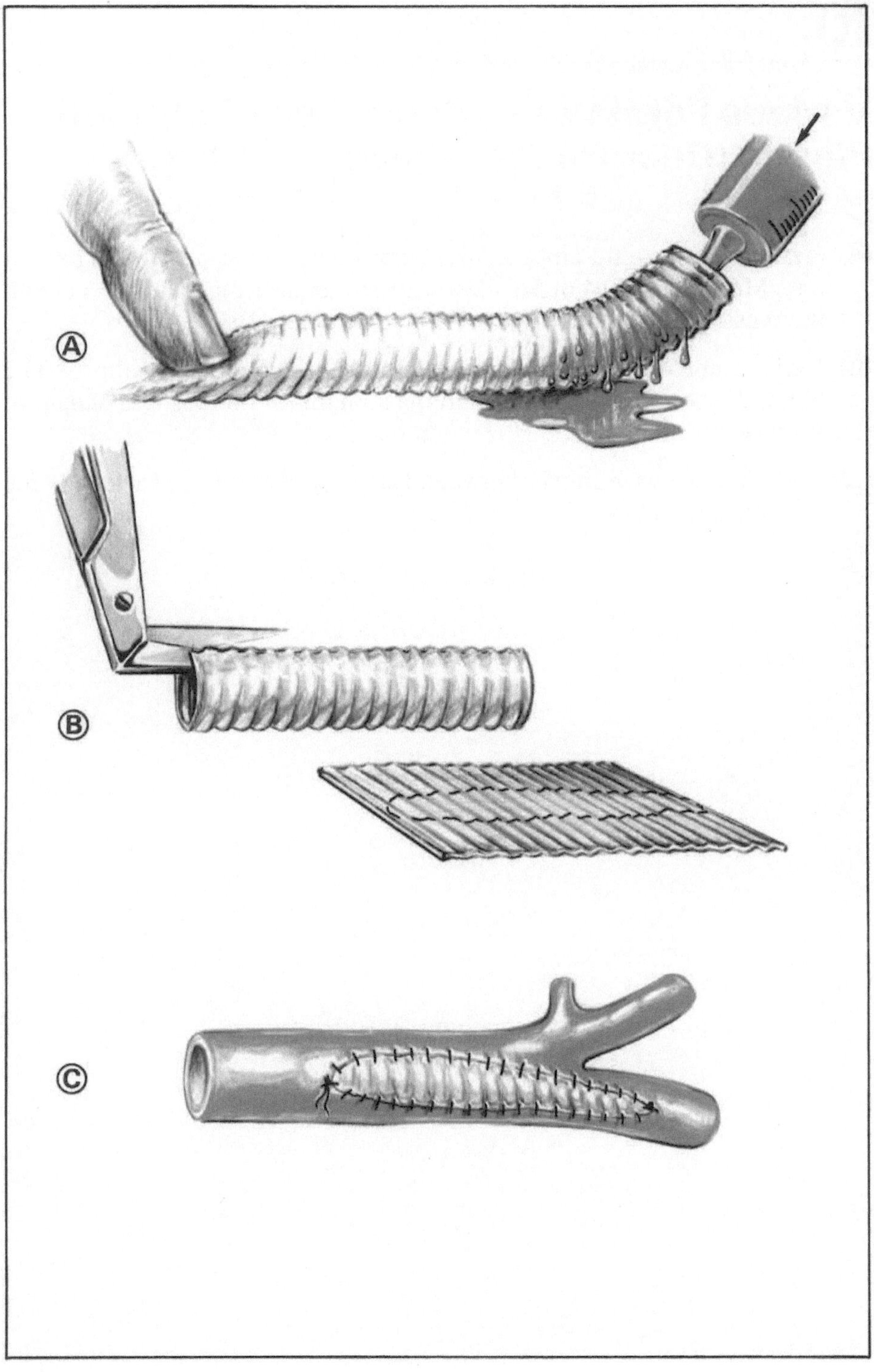

10

Various Forms of Anastomoses Between Plastic (Dacron) Prostheses and Arteries

Ⓐ Straight end-to-end anastomosis between a Dacron prosthesis and artery. Monofilament 4 or 5/0 plastic is used as suturing material. Technique basically the same as 4A–D.

Ⓑ Oblique end-to-end anastomosis. Suturing technique as above. The oblique anastomosis is safer than the straight for there is less danger of stenosis.

Ⓒ End-to-side anastomosis between Dacron prosthesis and artery. Same technique as 8A–D.

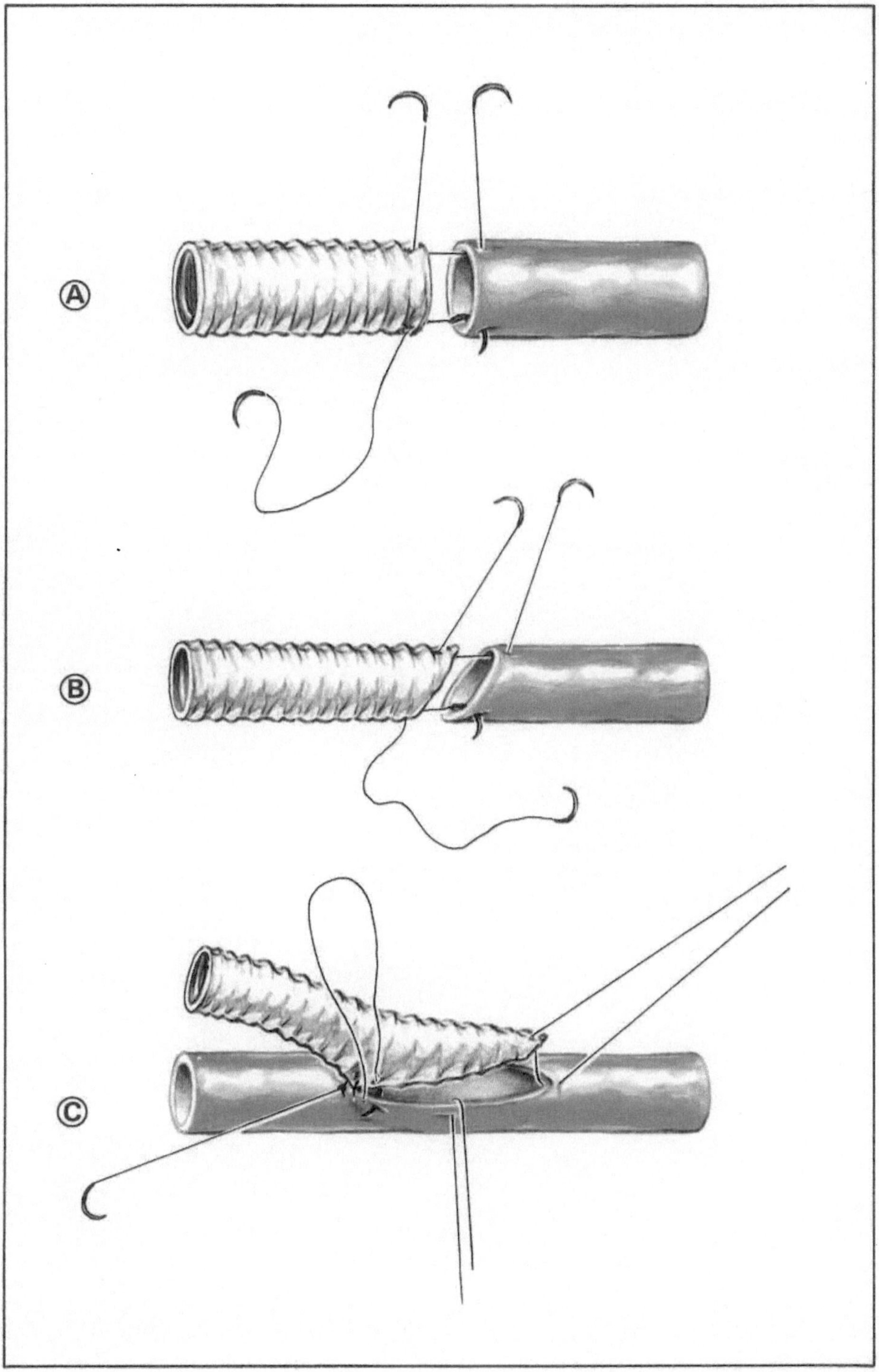

Typical Emergency Situations

11

Embolic Occlusion of the Right Common Femoral Artery at the Point of Bifurcation

Diagnostic Signs

Sudden onset, severe pain, peripheral ischemia, coldness, pallor, pulselessness. Later paresthesia and signs of paralysis. Embolic occlusion of the femoral bifurcation is the most common form of peripheral embolism (40% of all embolism). Aortic and iliac embolisms make up almost 20%. Just as the direct embolism of the femoral bifurcation, they are operated upon starting from the inguinal side. The same procedure as that which is described here applies to them as well. In the overwhelming majority of cases, preoperative angiography is not required.

Ⓐ Under local anesthesia (in younger patients with good circulatory conditions and low risk factors, general anesthesia may be used), the common femoral artery is exposed through a longitudinal incision in the inguinal region. If there is no pulse, the artery can be found by halving the length of the anterior iliac spine and its symphisis and making the incision distal to this halfway point.

The common femoral artery is prepared. The brownish-black thrombus can often be seen from the outside. The pulse ceases below the point of blockage.

Ⓑ A loop is placed around the bifurcation. This loop serves to allow control of bleeding. Thick, paraffin-coated silk thread or elastic rubber or plastic tubes are used for this.

Ⓐ

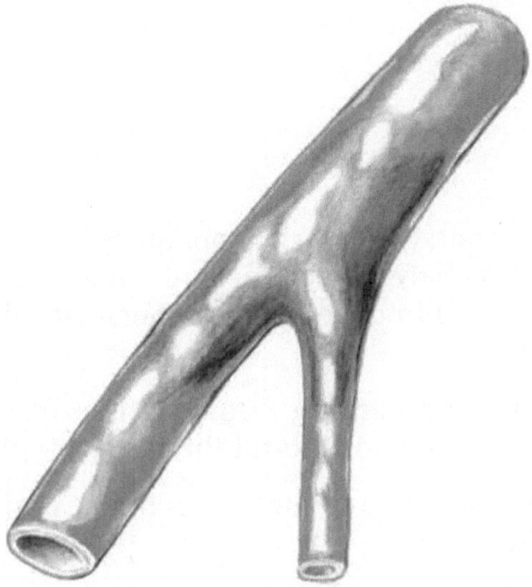

Ⓑ

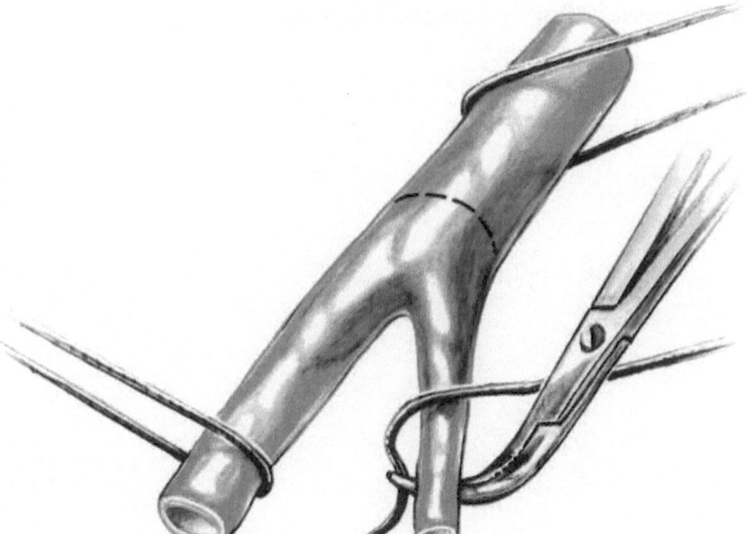

Important: Before opening the vessel, 5000 U heparin is administered intravenously to the patient.

Ⓒ The common femoral artery is cut obliquely. As a rule, the brownish-black embolism already projects forward somewhat. The Fogarty catheter No. 4 or No. 5 is introduced in a peripheral direction into the superficial femoral artery.

Ⓓ The embolism and separating thrombus is extracted with a Fogarty catheter. It is recommended to fill the Fogarty catheter with air.

This maneuver must be repeated several times until there is definite reflux from the vessel.

This reflux comes about as a result of rerouting the arterial blood through collaterals and it should be light red. However, it is often not very distinct and only becomes more abundant once blood has collected in the vessel after atraumatic clamping.

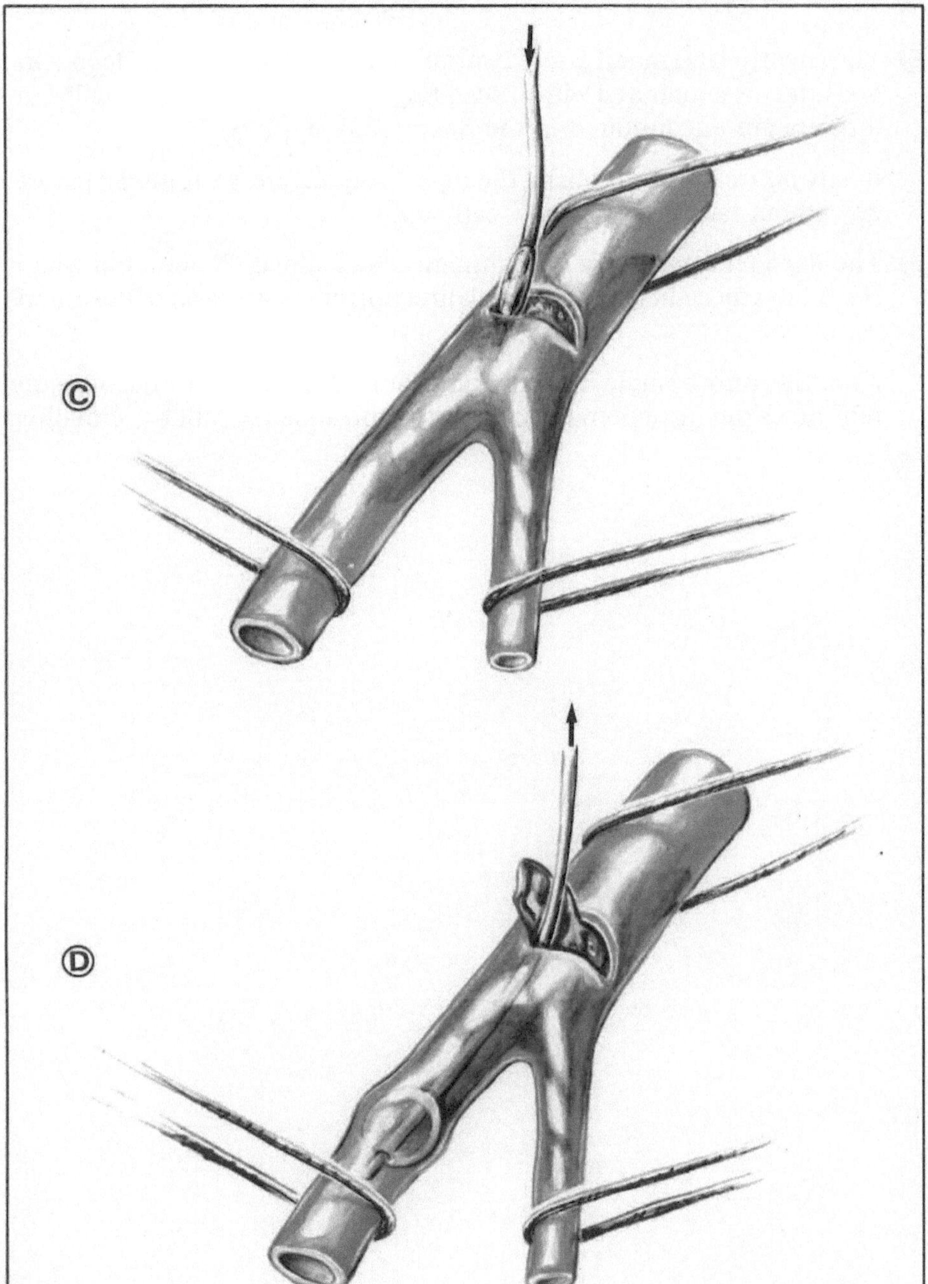
C
D

Ⓔ The superficial femoral artery is atraumatically clamped. The deep femoral artery is penetrated with a No. 4 Fogarty catheter. After some 15 cm, thrombi are encountered in the deep femoral artery.

In any bifurcation embolism, the deep femoral artery should be palpated without fail with a Fogarty catheter.

Ⓕ The deep femoral artery is atraumatically clamped. Penetration with a No. 5 Fogarty catheter in a central direction and extraction of the embolism.

As a rule, only a single maneuver is required since the arterial pressure reinforces the disobliterating measures and squeezes out the embolus.

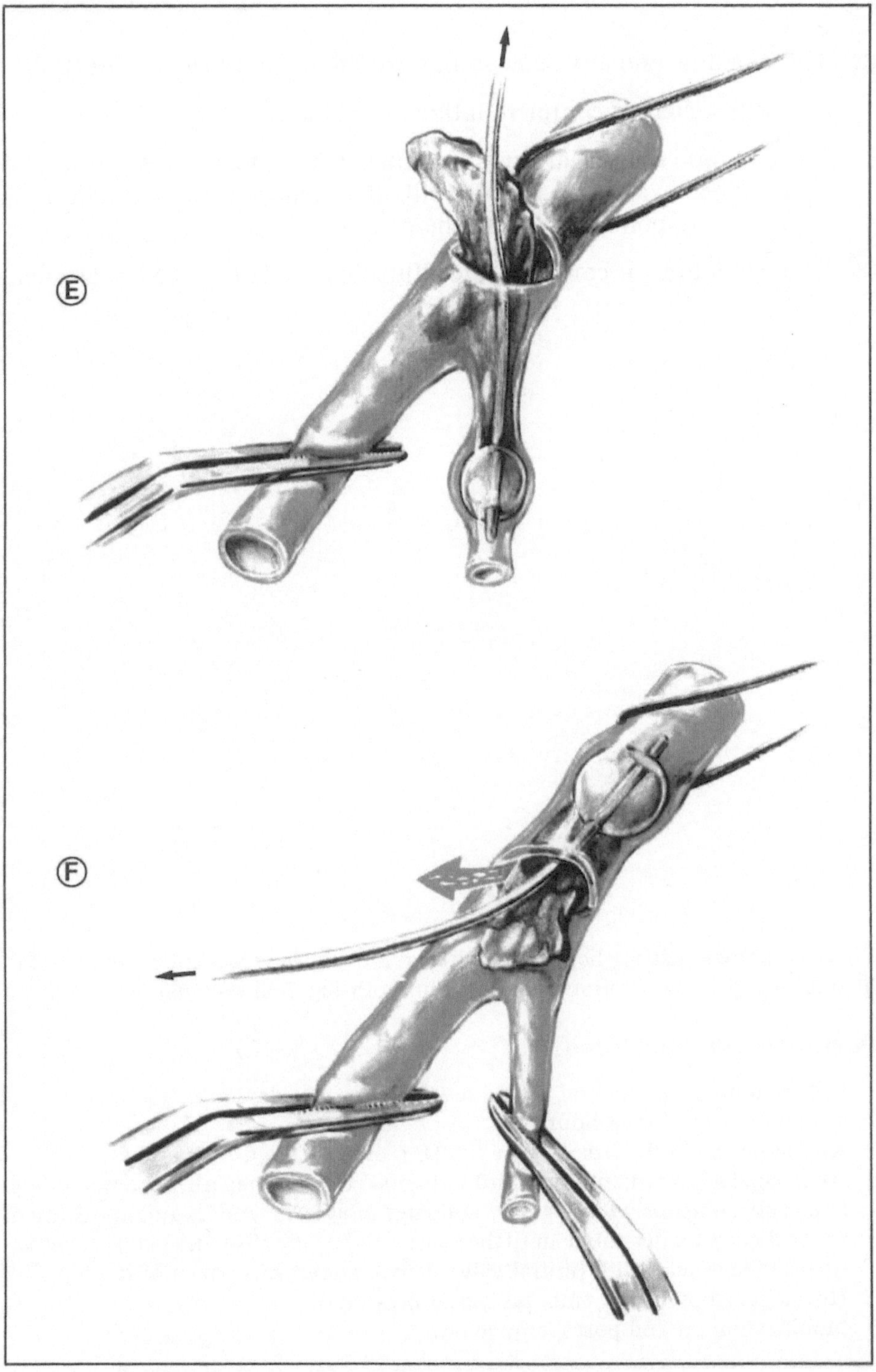
E
F

Ⓖ The embolus and any separating thrombi are completely removed.

The surest sign of complete inflow: it foams.

The common femoral artery is atraumatically clamped. A single continuous suture is started (5/0 monofilament plastic thread). Suturing is started at the point away from the operator.

Ⓗ The arteriotomy is complete after "flushing" and the thread is fastened.

This procedure is also applicable to indirect removal of an iliac embolism or embolism of the aortic bifurcation (starting from both inguinal regions).

Postoperative Measures

- Palpation of the peripheral pulses several times per day.
- Redon drainage for 48 hours.
- Antibiotic shield for 3 days with 2 x 2.0 g or 4 x 1.0 g Cefamandole.
- Anticoagulant treatment first with 3 to 4 x 5000 U depot-heparin per day administered subcutaneously for 3–4 days and later long-term anticoagulant treatment with a dicumarol derivative until the source of the embolism has been definitively traced and dealt with (mitral valve defect, aneurysms ahead of it, etc.).
- Histologic study of the embolus (atrial myxoma).
- Mobilization on 2nd postoperative day.

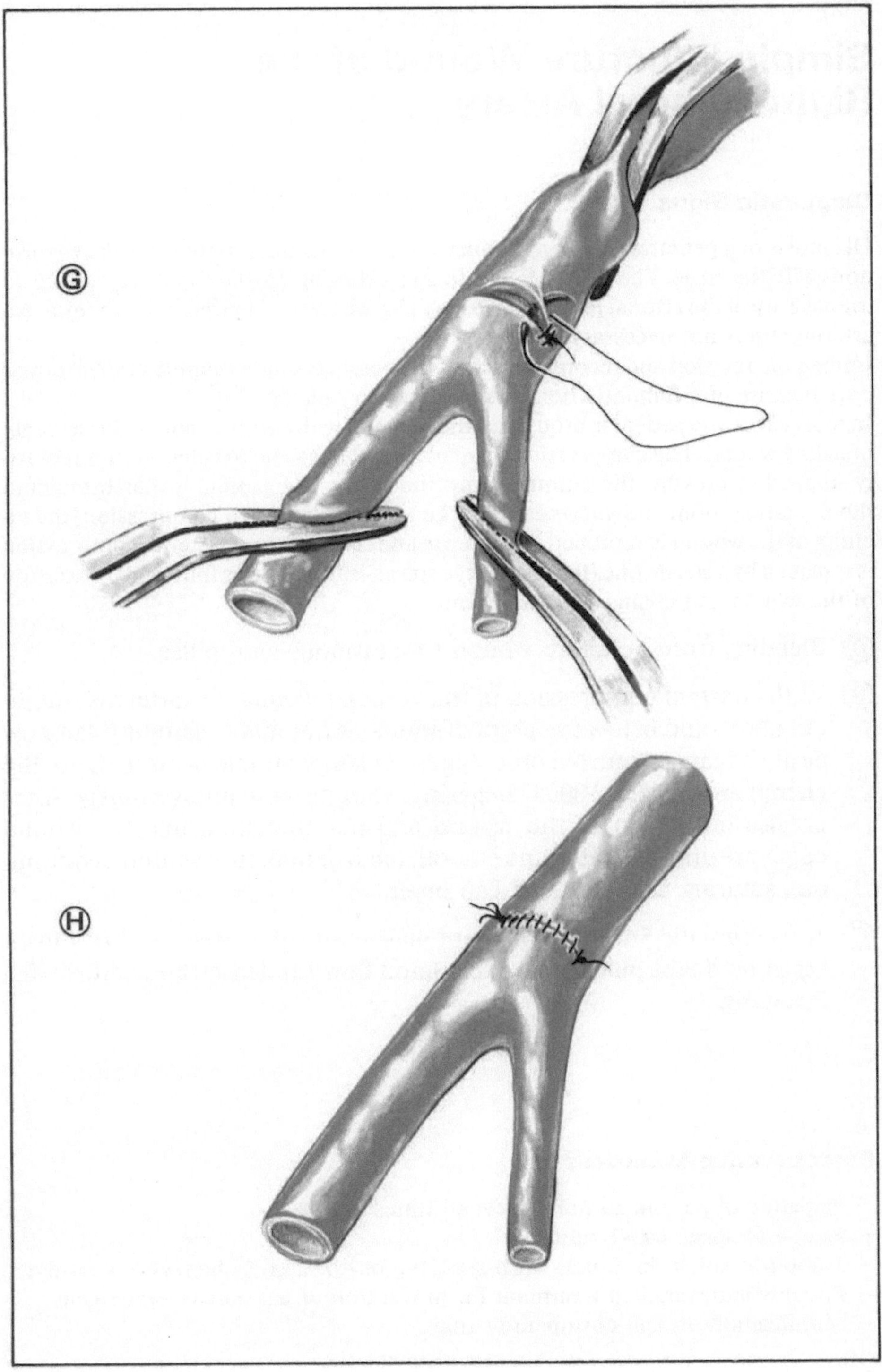
G
H

12

Simple Puncture Wound of the Right Femoral Artery

Diagnostic Signs

Diagnosis of a penetrating arterial injury is easy: bleeding is light red and synchronous with the pulse. The patient falls into an increasing state of shock. According to the severity of the arterial lesion, there may also be signs of peripheral ischemia. An arteriogram is not necessary.
Immediate revision and reconstruction of the vessel should be aimed at since nowadays ligature of a femoral artery is no longer acceptable.
In most cases, the patient is brought to the hospital with compression of the severely bleeding wound. The compression bandage is removed and the bleeding temporarily stopped by pressing the thumb against the artery. The patient is then brought to the operating room and anesthesia is begun. With continued compression, the vicinity of the wound is scrubbed until sterile and finally the non-sterile compression is replaced by a sterile one (for instance, a spone-stick). This is followed by excision of the wound and change of instruments.

Ⓐ Bleeding from puncture wound synchronous with pulse.

Ⓑ With constant compression of the vascular wound, the artery is sought out above and below the point of injury. Atraumatic clamping can now easily be carried out. No other types of clamps should be used. Once the clamps are in place, 5000 U heparin is administered intravenously. After precise inspection of the wound and determination that the wound edges are unremarkable and smooth (stab or puncture wound), continuous suturing of the wound can begin.

Ⓒ An atraumatic 5/0 monofilament plastic thread is used for this. Flushing should take place before the blood flow is released and before final fastening.

Postoperative Measures

- Palpation of peripheral pulses several times per day.
- Redon drainage for 48 hours.
- Antibiotic shield for 3 days with 2 x 2.0 g or 4 x 1.0 g Cefamandole per day.
- Possibly anticoagulant treatment for prevention of pulmonary embolisms.
- Mobilization on 2nd postoperative day.

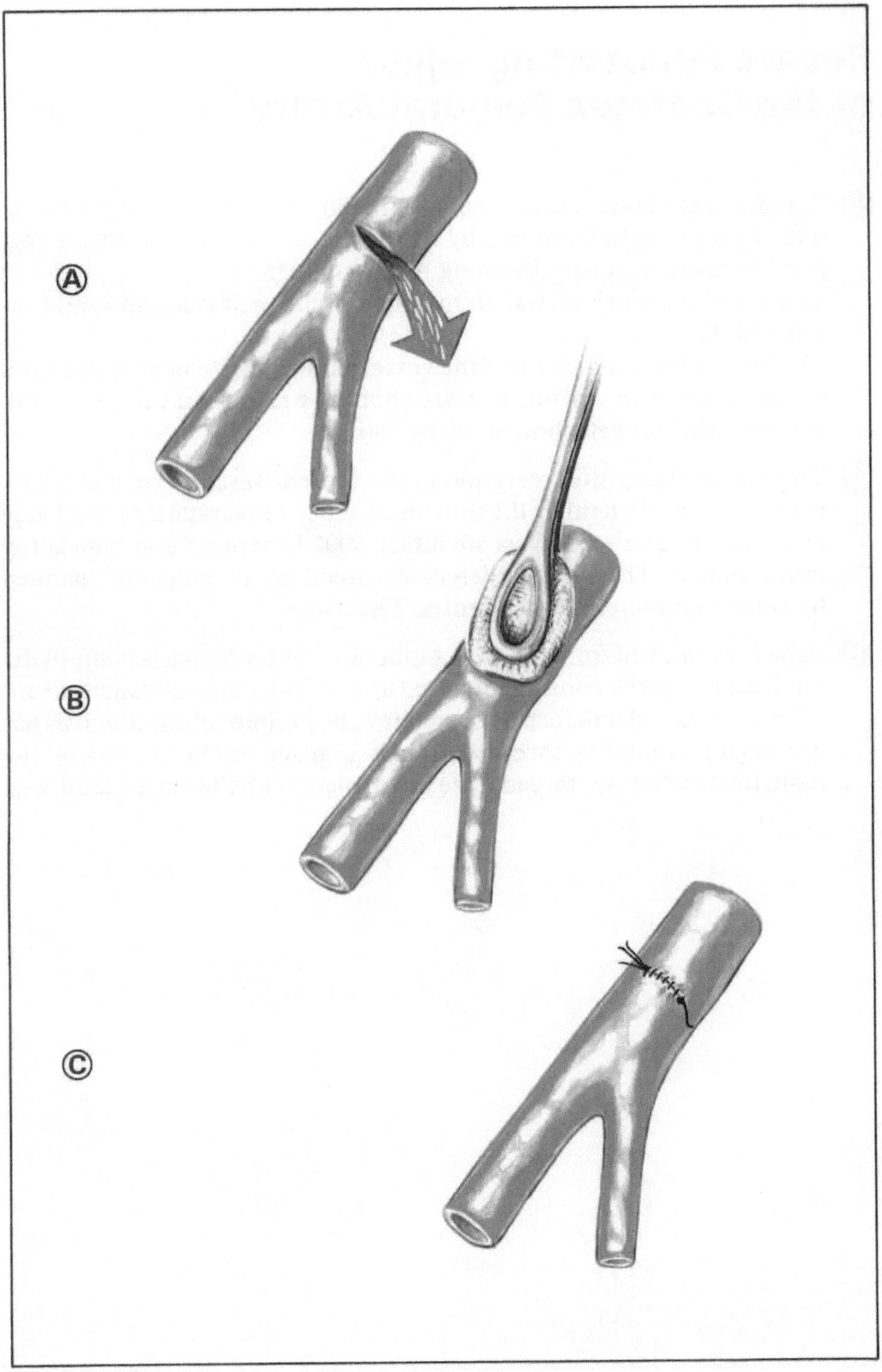

13

Severe Penetrating Injury of the Common Femoral Artery

Ⓐ The drawing shows a severe penetrating injury of the femoral bifurcation, such as might be caused by a shot: the edges of the vessel are ragged and there is severe bleeding to the outside.
The vessel, meanwhile, was atraumatically clamped in a central and peripheral direction.
The broken lines indicate that the vessel stumps had to be resected until a healthy segment was found. Care should be taken that the vessel wall is intact with no detachment of the intima.

Ⓑ This shows status after resection of the injured vascular segment. The vessel stumps are held by the threads of a loop to counteract a tendency to retraction. The wall layers are intact. 5000 U heparin is administered intravenously. The vascular defect produced can no longer be spanned by simple end-to-end anastomosis. Therefore,

Ⓒ a piece is removed from the great saphenous vein which is usually of the same caliber as the common femoral artery. This piece of vein is inserted into the vascular defect. In the picture the peripheral anastomosis has just begun. A holding thread is already in place on the left and on the right, the two "corner threads" are put in place with the usual technique.

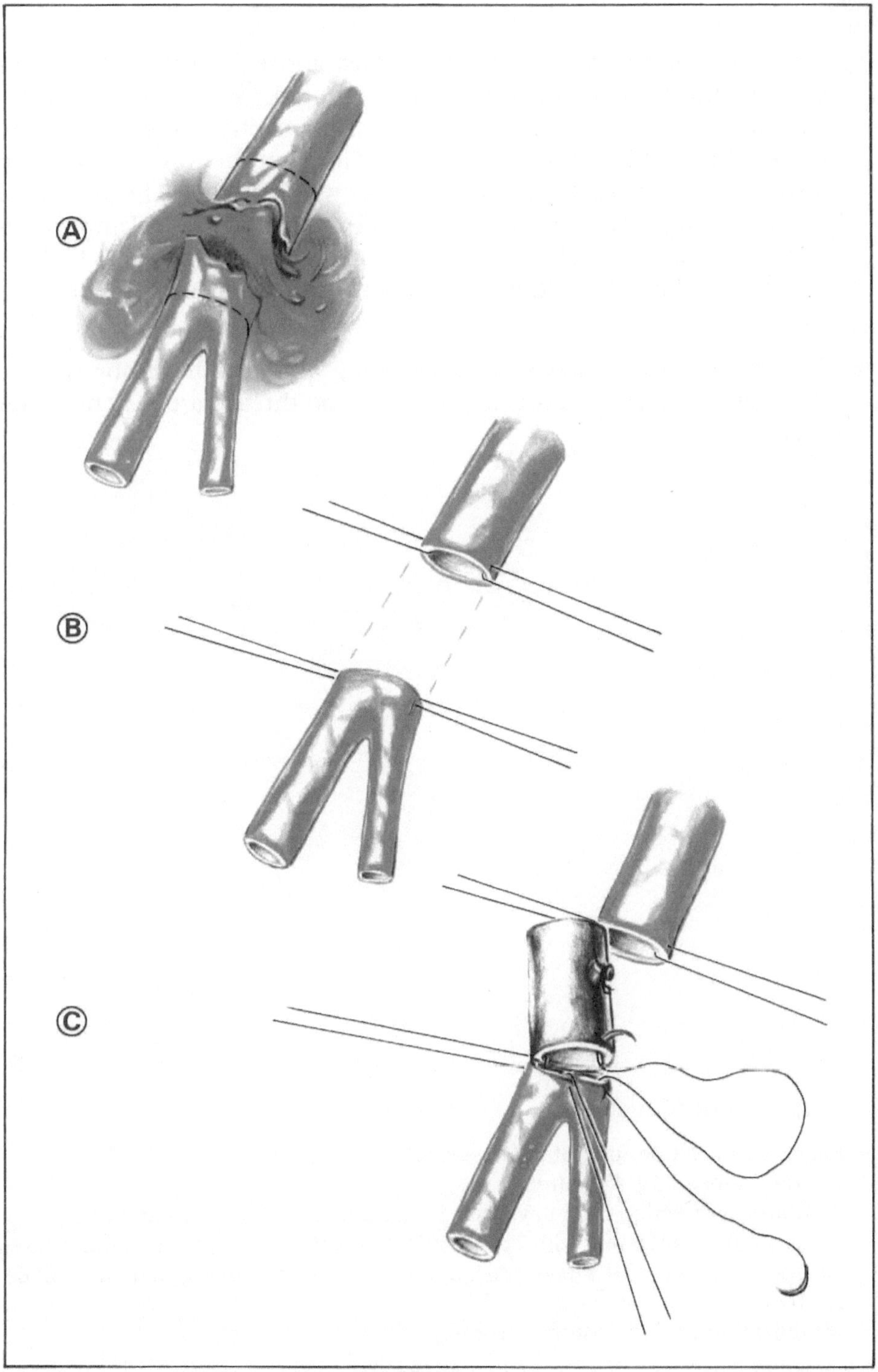

Ⓓ The posterior wall of the peripheral anastomosis between the piece of vein and the peripheral vessel stump is sutured. (When, as in this case, "turning" of the anastomosis is not possible owing to the bifurcation, the vessel must be sutured from the inside, but care must be taken to fasten on the outside). Next, the anterior wall is started. The peripheral atraumatic vascular clamps are removed and one of these clamps is placed on the piece of vein above the completed anastomosis, so that the suture can close. Next, the central anastomosis is made with the same technique.

Ⓔ Status after reconstruction of a penetrating wound of the femoral artery. The central anastomosis is completed. The threads are fastened after flushing.

Postoperative Measures

- Palpation of the peripheral pulse several times per day.
- Redon drainage for 48 hours.
- Antibiotic protection for 5 days with 3 x 2.0 g or 6 x 1.0 g Cefamandole per day.
- Anticoagulant treatment with 3 to 4 x 5000 U depot-heparin per day administered subcutaneously for 3 - 4 days. It is not necessary to continue with dicumarol derivatives.
- Mobilization on 3rd postoperative day.

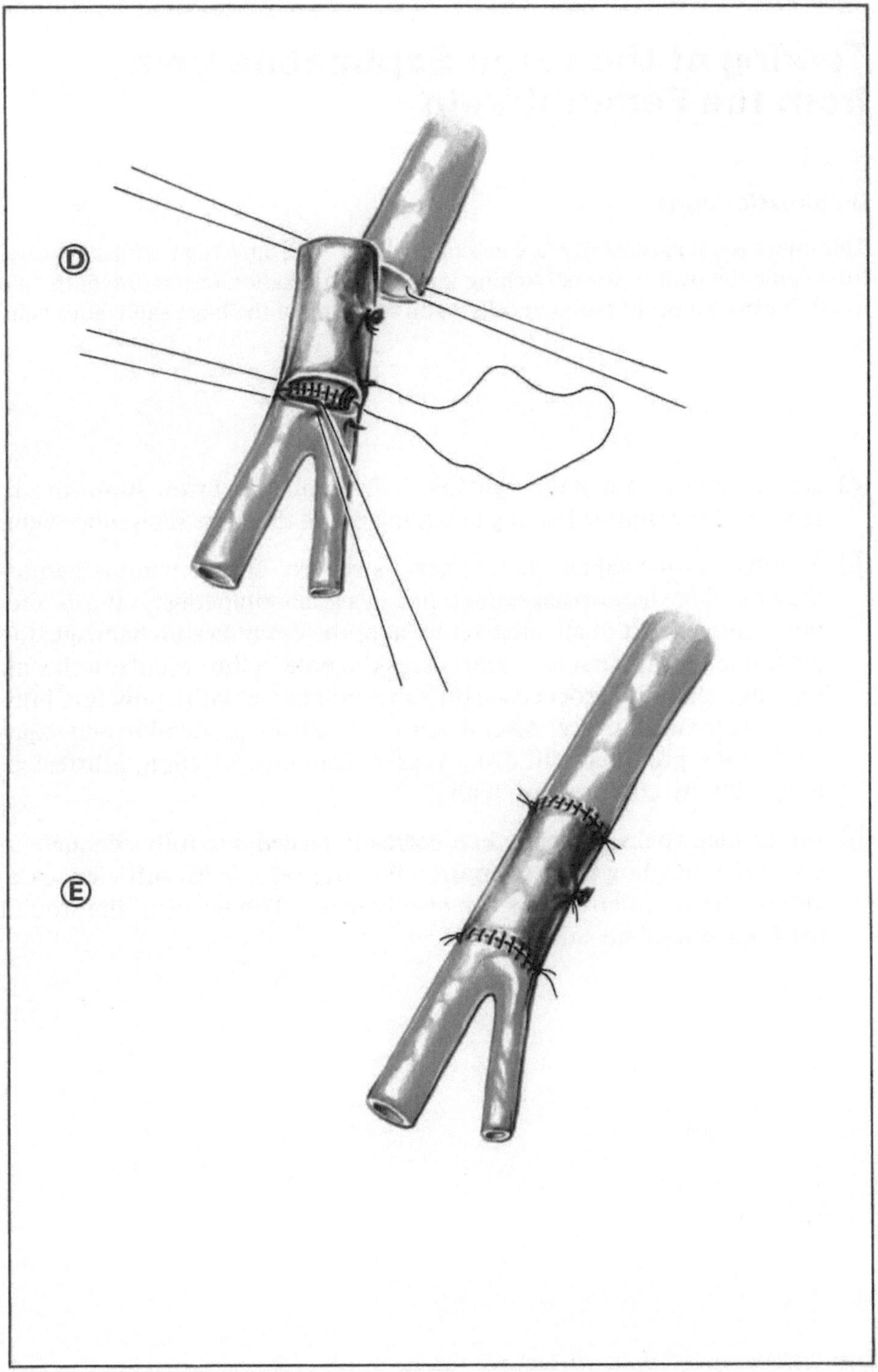
D
E

14

Tearing of the Large Saphenous Vein from the Femoral Vein

Diagnostic Signs

This injury is not particularly rare and occurs in severe, open hip traumas (injuries from being run over or overstretching injuries with luxation or fracture of the hip joint). It can also occur iatrogenically upon stripping of the large saphenous vein.

Ⓐ Anatomic situation in the right inguinal region. The arrow shows the direction of the trauma leading to tearing out of the large saphenous vein.

Ⓑ Tearing out has taken place. There is severe, diffuse venous hemorrhaging. The hemorrhage does not cease spontaneously and is life-threatening. First of all, after removal of the compression bandage, the person rendering first aid compresses the hole in the vascular wall with a sponge-stick and proceeds in the same manner as with a puncture injury of the femoral artery. After dealing with the local situation and exposure of the proximal and distal vessel segments, bleeding is arrested, preferably by compression with

Ⓒ two sponge-sticks, which, when correctly placed, are fully adequate to arrest the bleeding from an injured femoral vein. With sufficient care, atraumatic vascular clamps can also be used. The edges of the wound are then smoothed out.

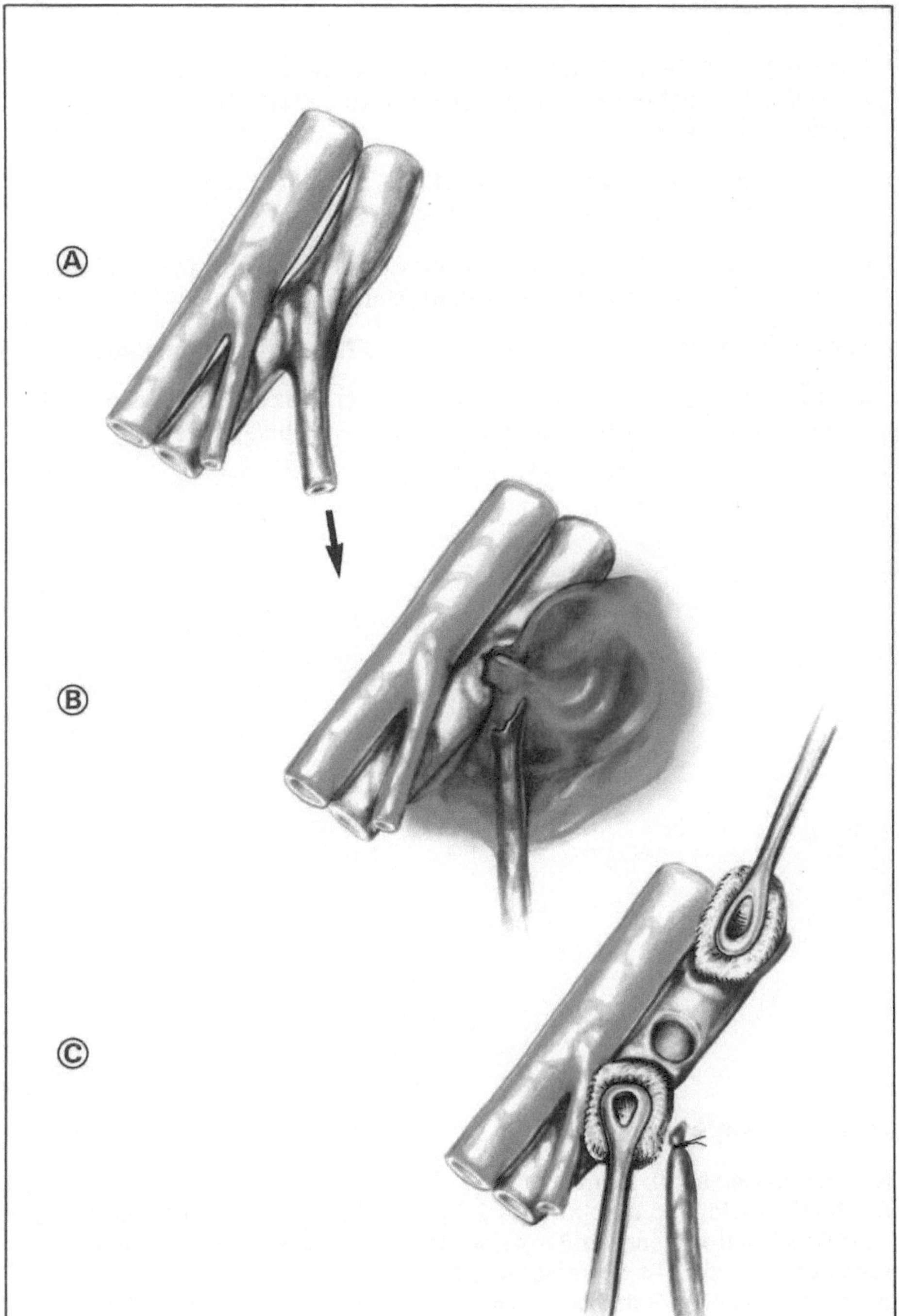

Ⓓ If the defect in the wall oft the vein is not to large (up to half the circumference), direct oblique suturing may be attempted, although not infrequently it leads to

Ⓔ stenosis, as shown in this picture. If a larger defect is produced in the wall of the vein, we recommend the use of

Ⓕ a venous patch, taken from the periphery. Often the proximal end piece of the torn out large saphenous vein is suitable for this.

Sewing in the venous patch is no more difficult than direct suturing.

Suturing takes place according to the same criteria as the suturing technique of a venous patch on an artery, as described earlier.

Postoperative Measures

- Redon drainage for 48 hours.
- Antibiotic shield for 5 days with 3 x 2.0 g or 6 x 1.0 g Cefamandole for 5 days.
- Anticoagulant treatment with 3 to 4 x 5000 U depot-heparin per day administered subcutaneously for 3–4 days, followed by
- change to a dicumarol derivative, administered for at least a further 6 months.
- Bandaging and elevation of the leg.
- Mobilization on the 3rd postoperative day, early active and passive exercises.

D

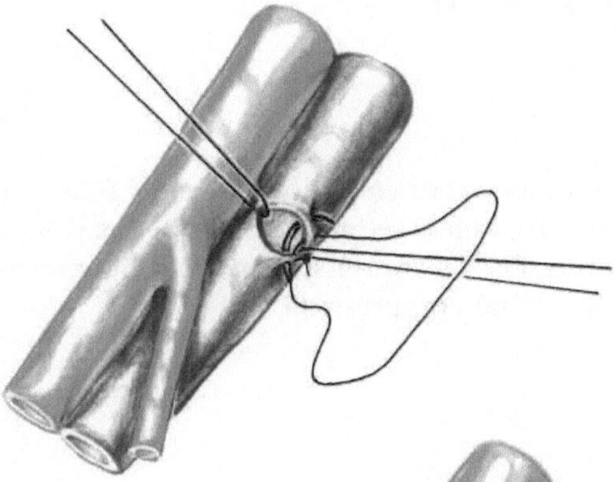

E

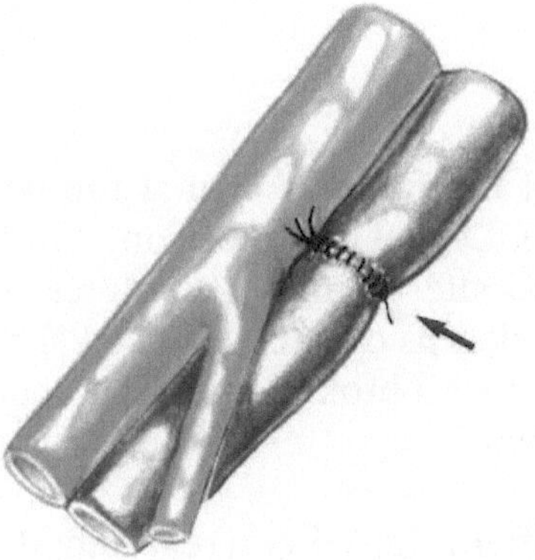

F

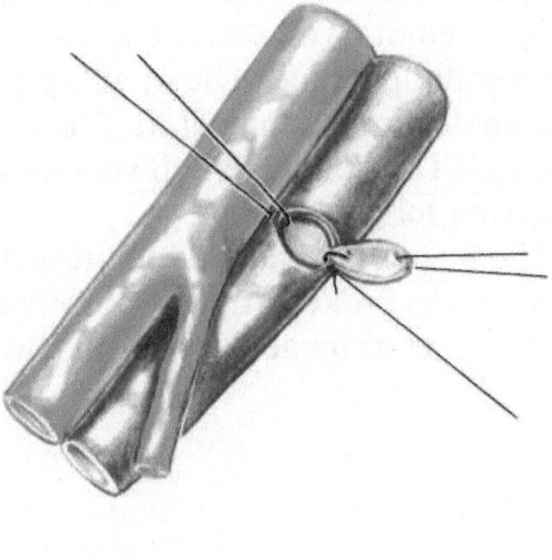

15

Severe Penetrating Injury of the Common Femoral Vein

Diagnostic Signs

Profuse venous bleeding, patient in severe condition of shock. Bleeding does not stop spontaneously since the mechanism of retraction of the vessel stumps does not exist in veins as it does in arteries. Person administering first aid removes the compression bandage and attempts digital compression.

Ⓐ Penetrating injury of the femoral vein at the point of opening of the great saphenous vein. Digital compression. After exposure of the vein above and below the site of injury, compression with sponge-stick. Atraumatic vascular clamps can also be used. The lines of the planned resection are drawn in with broken lines. Resection must take place far in the healthy segment.

Ⓑ Injured vascular segments have been resected, the common and superficial femoral veins have been atraumatically clamped, direct anastomosis is not possible. The opening portion of the large saphenous vein is prepared for vascular graft. The distal stump of the saphenous vein is ligated. The double length venous segment, which is to be used as graft, is split longitudinally.
The planned oblique line of resection of the piece of saphenous vein is shown by broken lines for construction of a composite replacement vessel, so as to be able to obtain the necessary caliber.

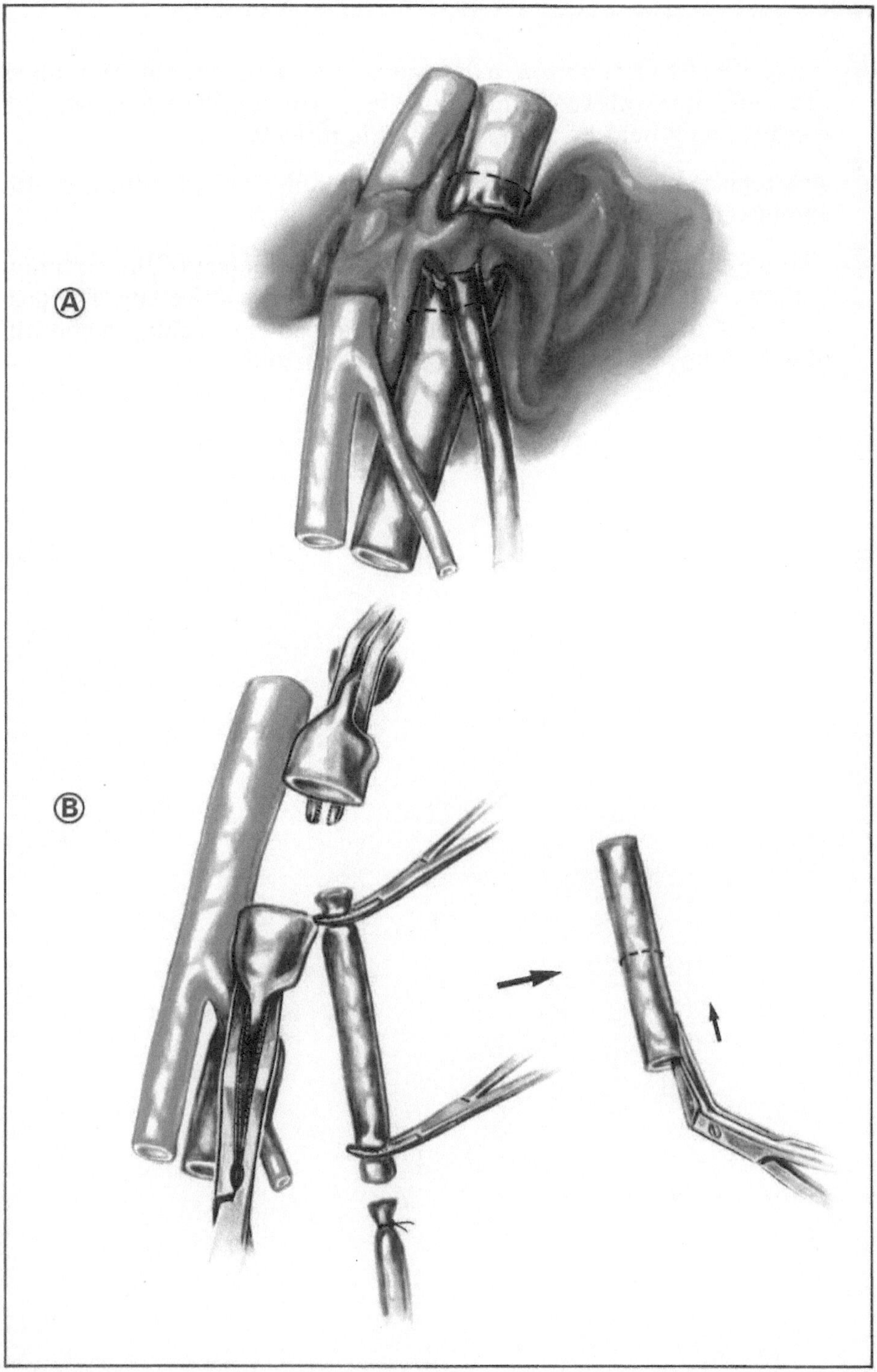

Ⓒ The piece of vein cut through the middle is anastomosed in the manner of a door hinge with a continuous suture (5/0 monofilament thread), the corners being held by means of holding threads.

Ⓓ The replacement vessel is completed, the other row of sutures is also completed.

Ⓔ The peripheral anastomosis in the area of the defect of the common femoral vein is completed, the atraumatic clamp is moved up. The posterior wall of the upper anastomosis has already been sutured and will now be followed by suturing of the anterior wall.

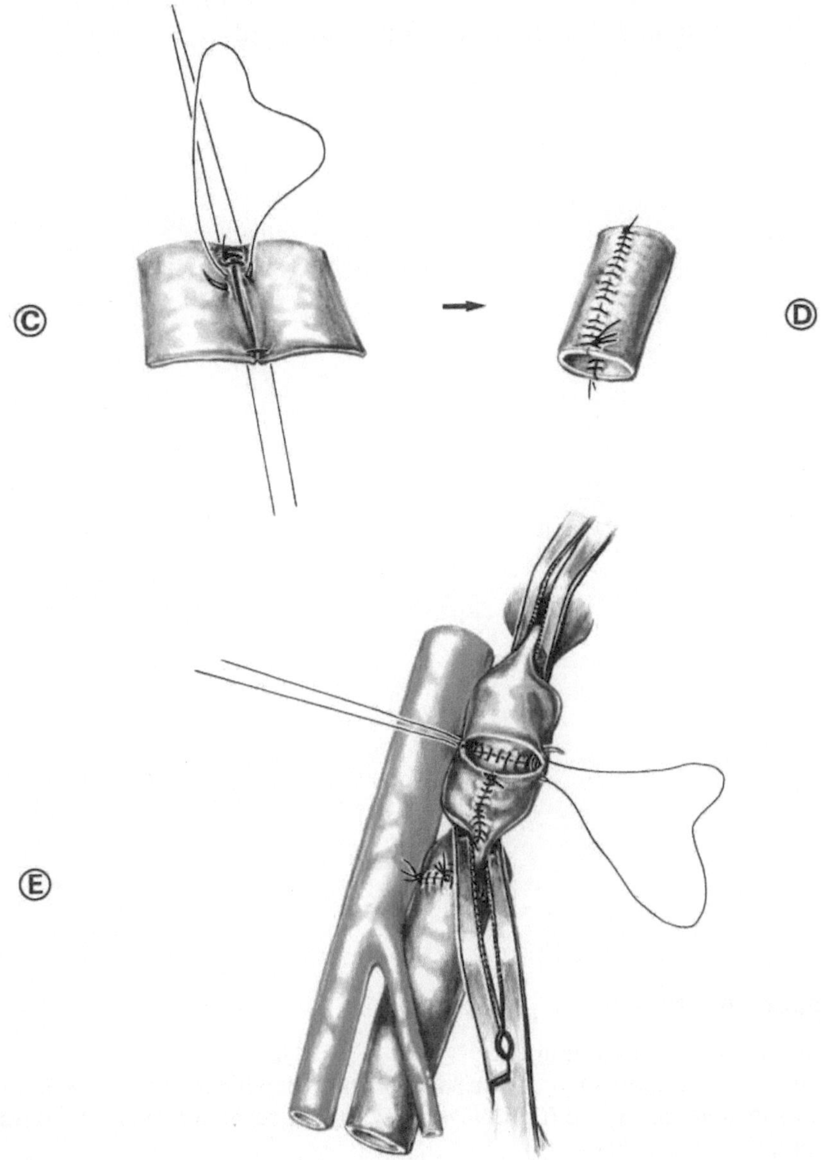

Ⓕ After flushing, the threads of the proximal anastomosis of the venous graft are fastened. Reconstruction is completed.

Postoperative Measures

- Redon drainage for 48 hours.
- Anticoagulant treatment, first with 3 to 4 x 5000 U depot heparin per day administered subcutaneously and from the 4th day, a dicumarol derivative for at least 6 months.
- Antibiotic shield for 3–5 days with 3 x 2.0 g or 6 x 1.0 g Cefamandole per day.
- Active and passive leg exercises to promote venous blood flow and prevention of postoperative thrombosis.
- Close bandage on the operated extremity to promote blood flow to the deep leg veins and elevation of the limb.
- Mobilization on 3rd postoperative day.

Ⓕ

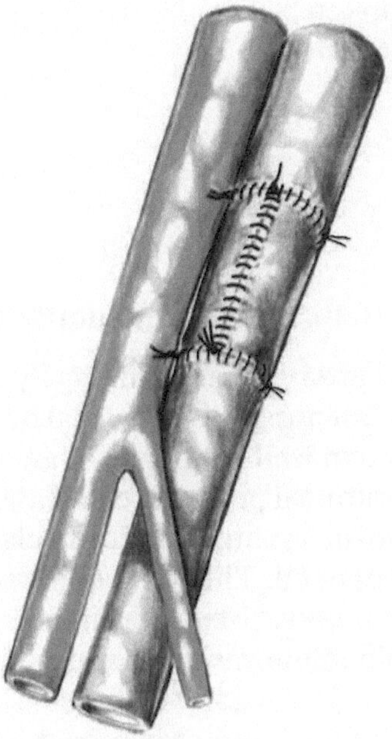

16

False Aneurysm of the Common Femoral Artery

Diagnostic Signs

Status after direct vascular trauma (such as after a stab injury, an earlier vascular operation or vascular puncture, etc.). Pulsating, growing, painful tumor in the groin. No signs of peripheral ischemia.

Ⓐ Pulsating hematoma (false aneurysm) shortly before rupture.

Ⓑ The common femoral artery ise atraumatically clamped above the pulsating tumor. If this is not possible for tactical or anatomical reasons, the external iliac artery is exposed by means of an incision in the lower abdomen with a retroperitoneal procedure and after intravenous administration of 5000 U heparin, it is atraumatically clamped. Next, the wall of the false aneurysm is opened. The wall consists of hematomatous masses and pseudomembranous tissue formations. There is fairly severe bleeding from the hole in the vascular wall, which can best be stopped with a Fogarty catheter. The Fogarty catheter is introduced into the hole in the vascular wall, inflated and drawn back. This obviates time-consuming preparation of the distal vessels.

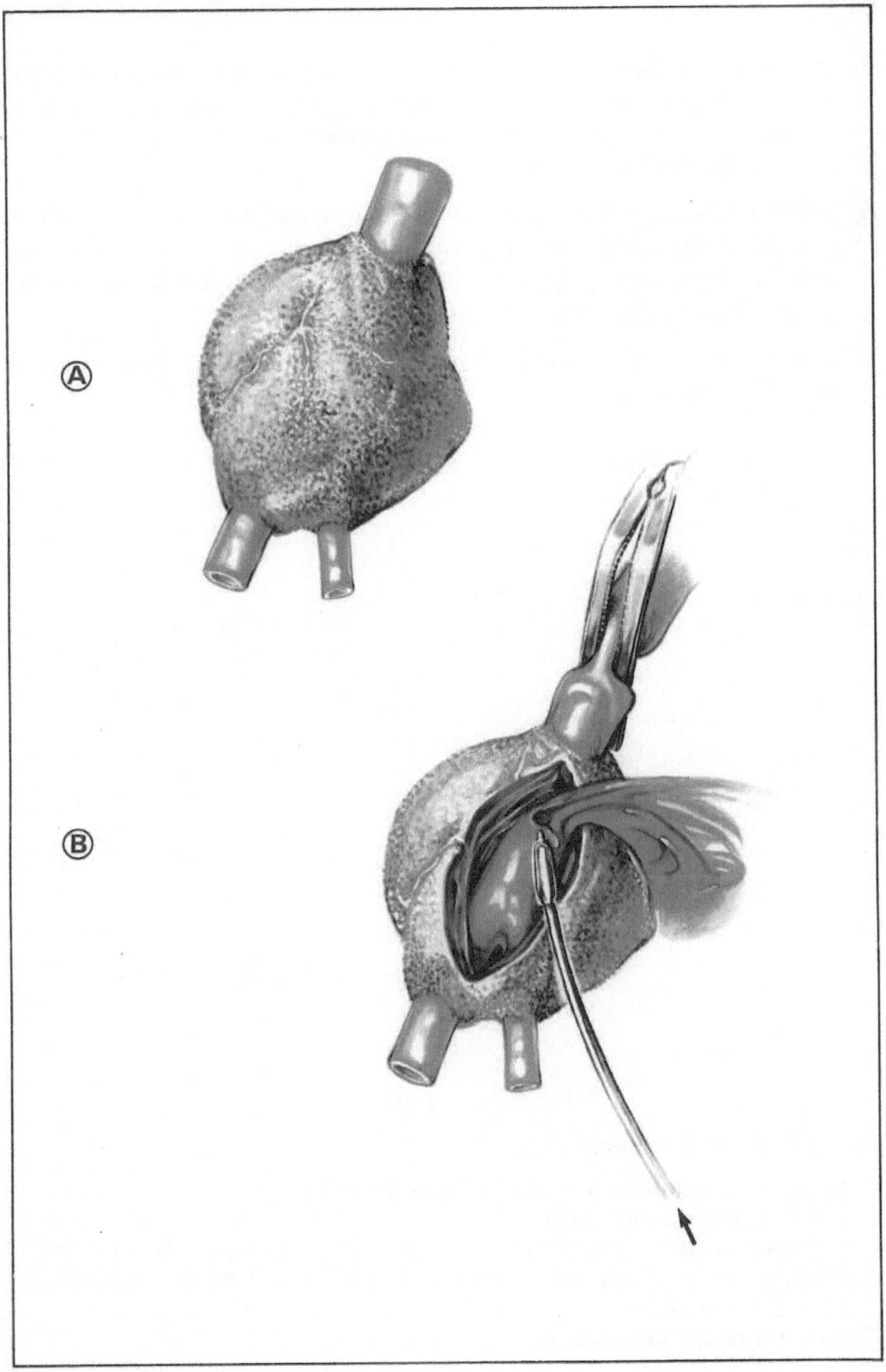

Ⓒ The common femoral artery or the external iliac artery are clamped on the central side, reflux bleeding is blocked by the inflated, drawn back Fogarty catheter. The hematoma is now completely cleared out so as to avoid wound infection later.

Ⓓ After clearing out the hematoma, an atraumatic clamp is placed at the peripheral end and the Fogarty catheter is removed. In most cases, the defect in the vascular wall can be closed with a simple X or U suture with an atraumatic monofilament thread.

Ⓔ Status after sewing up the hole in the vascular wall and elimination of the false aneurysm.

Postoperative Measures

- Peripheral palpation of the pulse, several times per day.
- Redon drainage for 48 hours.
- Antibiotic shield for 3 days with 2 x 2.0 g or 4 x 1.0 g Cefamandole per day.
- Anticoagulant treatment with heparin only in patients at risk for prevention of pulmonary embolism.
- Mobilization on 2nd postoperative day.

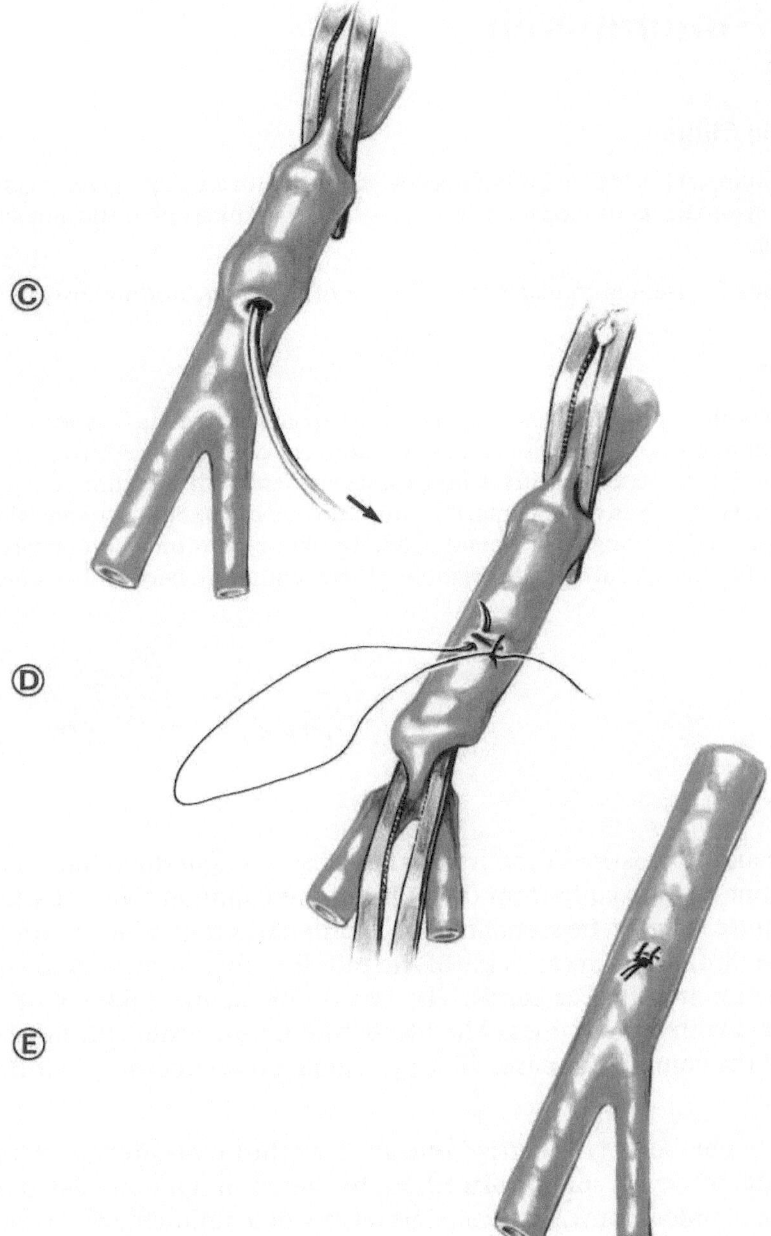

C
D
E

17

Thrombectomy of the Right Femoral Vein

Diagnostic Signs

Marked swelling of the leg with bluish discoloration, relatively slight pain. Pressure pain in the inguinal region and along the course of the femoral vein on the inner side of the thigh.

Phlebography is essential to disclose the extent of the venous thrombosis.

Indication

Operation is only appropriate within 7 days of the appearance of the first symptoms of venous thrombosis. Fibrinolytic treatment should be considered. As a rule, however, fibrinolysis is not possible in freshly operated patients. An operation is only indicated if there are signs of phlegmasia cerulea dolens in younger patients with a varying degree of swelling to prevent a post thrombotic syndrome and in case of loose thrombi washed out by phlebography to prevent pulmonary embolisms.

Ⓐ Status after exposure of the femoral vein by a longitudinal incision in the groin just medially from the pulse of the common femoral artery. The entire leg must be scrubbed until sterile, so as to be able to squeeze out the thrombi from the veins of the calf. For this, it is best to prepare sterile Esmarch rubber bands. The line of the planned phlebotomy is drawn in with broken lines. The black thrombus is visible through the wall of the vein. In this case, the large saphenous vein is not yet thrombosed.

Ⓑ Oblique phlebotomy is carried out. A black thrombus protrudes from the phlebotomy. A loop is placed on the common femoral vein above the site of phlebotomy. Care must be taken not to injure the deep femoral vein, which opens into the common femoral vein in this region. Sparing preparation of the common femoral vein is recommended so as to prevent later shrinkage of scars or renewed phlebothrombosis.

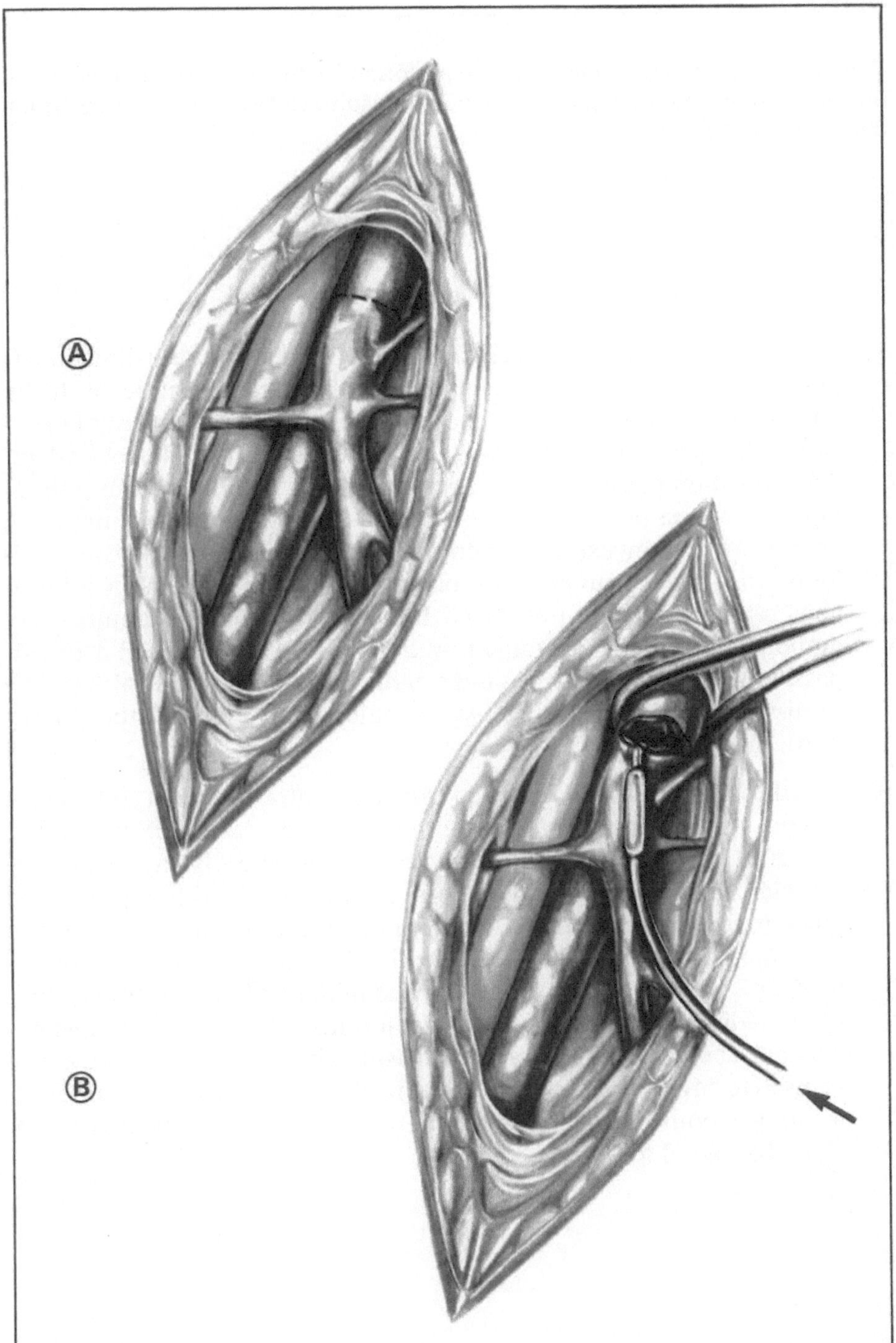

Venous thrombectomy should never be performed without prior determination of the blood group and placing banked blood in readiness. Use of an autotransfusion pump may also be appropriate.

Ⓒ The No. 6 or 8 Fogarty catheter, pushed forward in a central direction, is pulled back in the inflated state and the thrombus is extracted. If the operation is performed under local anesthesia, the patient should activate abdominal pressure (Valsalva's maneuver), or if it is performed under intubation anesthesia, the anesthetist must apply artificial respiration with excess pressure so as to prevent the possibility of a pulmonary embolism. The measure formerly used of introducing a "closing balloon" positioned from the contralateral side and inflated in the inferior vena cava is no longer necessary. It has been found that a pulmonary embolism cannot be prevented by this means. However, an active or passive Valsalva maneuver is important. The patient should also be in a semi-seated position during the operation (anti-Trendelenburg position).

Ⓓ The thrombus has been removed from the central direction and there is a good, respiration-dependent venous flow. The central portion of the common femoral vein is blocked with a sponge-stick. Next, the Fogarty catheter is introduced in a peripheral direction and an attempt must be made to lead the catheter past the venous valves by means of twisting movements. The leg is kept elevated by the assistant and an attempt is made, by smoothing out, squeezing and milking of the extremity, to remove additional thrombi from the deep veins of the calf. These maneuvers must be repeated several times. Esmarch rubber bands should also be used to "milk" the extremity. When all thrombi have been removed, a strong venous inflow emerges. There is the possibility of a fairly considerable blood loss.

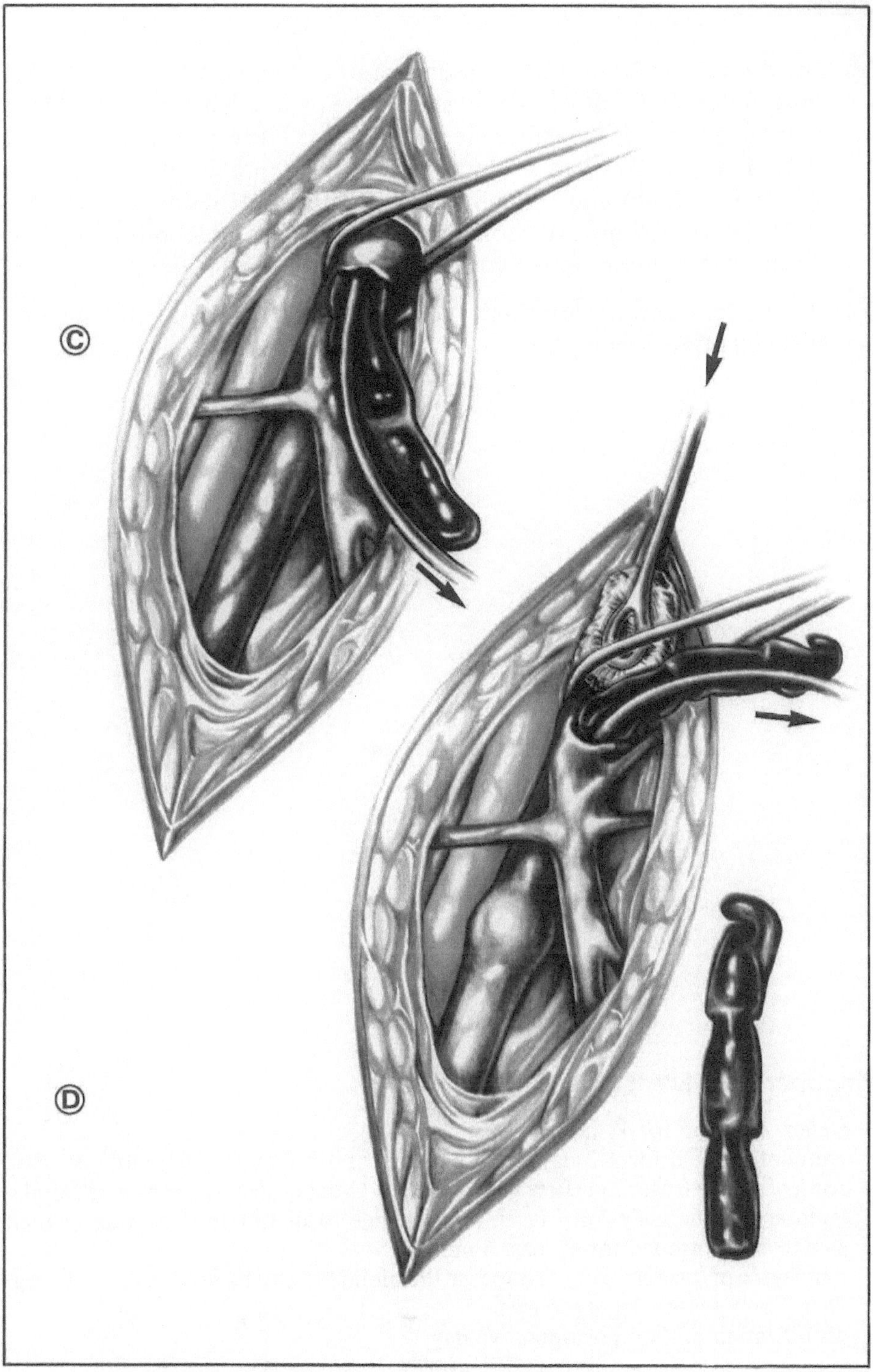
C
D

Ⓔ The thrombi are removed from the peripheral and central side and venous blood flows out from both sides. The patient has received 5000 U heparin intravenously before the phlebotomy. The efferent and afferent parts of the femoral vein are compressed with a sponge-stick or blocked by careful atraumatic "step-by-step" clamping. Holding threads are sewn into the corners of the phlebotomy and the phlebotomy is then closed with a continuous suture (5/0 monofilament thread).

Ⓕ Status after thrombectomy and suturing of the phlebotomy (thread only fastened after flushing).

Postoperative Measures

- Redon drainage for 48 hours.
- Antibiotic shield for 2–3 days with 2 x 2.0 g or 4 x 1.0 g Cefamandole per day.
- Anticoagulant treatment, first with 4 x 5000 U depot-heparin per day administered subcutaneously for 4 days, then change to dicumarol treatment, which should be continued for at least 6 months.
- Bandaging of the extremity to increase the blood flow to the deep veins of the leg.
- Active and passive leg exercises.
- Mobilization on 2nd postoperative day.

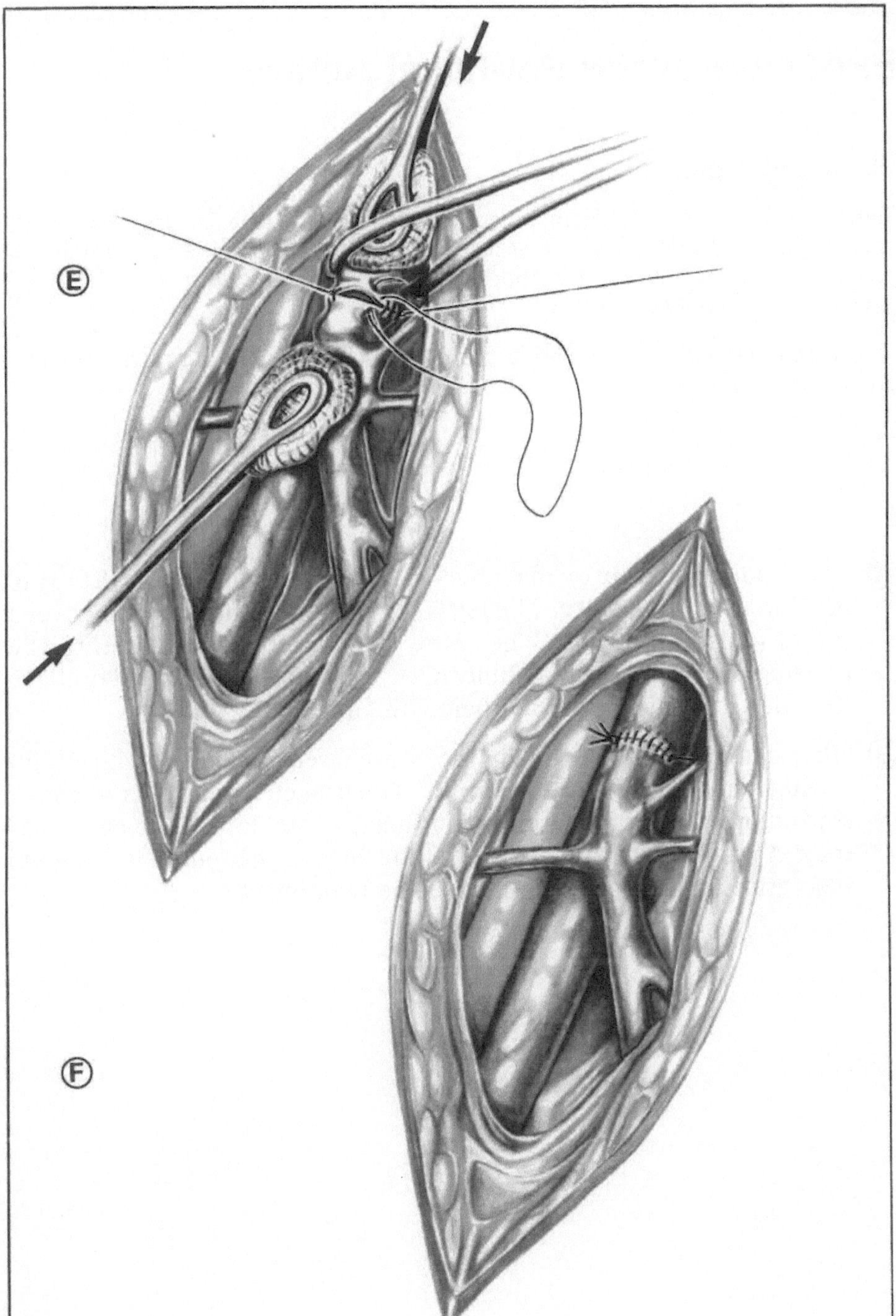
E
F

18

Exposure of the Popliteal Artery

Diagnostic Signs

Signs of acute peripheral ischemia. Femoral pulse readily palpable. In patients who are not adipose, the pulse can also be palpated on the thigh over the course of the superficial femoral artery. On the other hand, the pulse of the popliteal artery is not palpable in the popliteal space.

Suspicion of embolic or thrombotic obstruction of the popliteal artery. Angiography is required.

Ⓐ Longitudinal incision on the inner side of the head of the tibia in the upper third of the lower leg. The leg is lightly bent at the knee joint over a pad or folded scrub shirt. The entire leg is scrubbed until sterile. The drawing also shows the possibility of exposing the popliteal artery above the knee joint by an incision below the adductor canal.

Ⓑ After cutting through the skin, the crural fascia is exposed with the inserting tendons of the pes anserinus. The broken line shows the line of separation of the crural fascia, including the 3 tendons of the pes anserinus. At bottom right in the picture, the large saphenous vein is shown held aside, which must, at all costs, be kept intact.

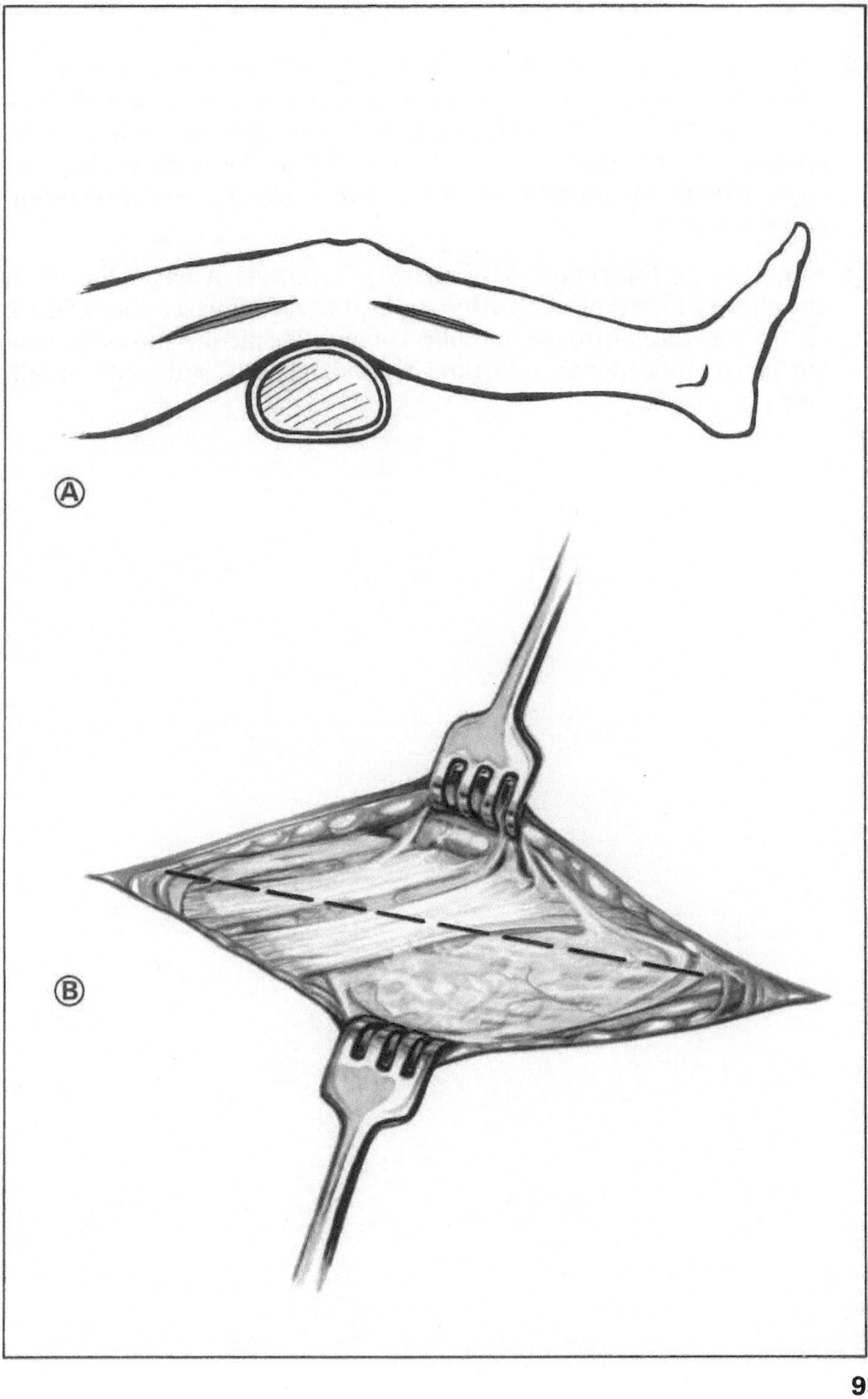

Ⓒ After severing the crural fascia, cutting through the pes anserinus and retraction of the medial portion of the gastrocnemium muscle, the vascular nerve bundle of the popliteal space comes into view. In front is the tibial nerve and part of the popliteal vein. Behind these, the popliteal artery is visible. It is connected to the popliteal vein by a very close vascular septum.

Ⓓ After severing this common vascular septum between the popliteal vein and artery, a loop is placed on the popliteal artery, which is made of thick paraffin-coated silk thread or rubber tubing. The picture shows the popliteal artery looped with a silk thread, the tibial nerve and popliteal vein being held aside.

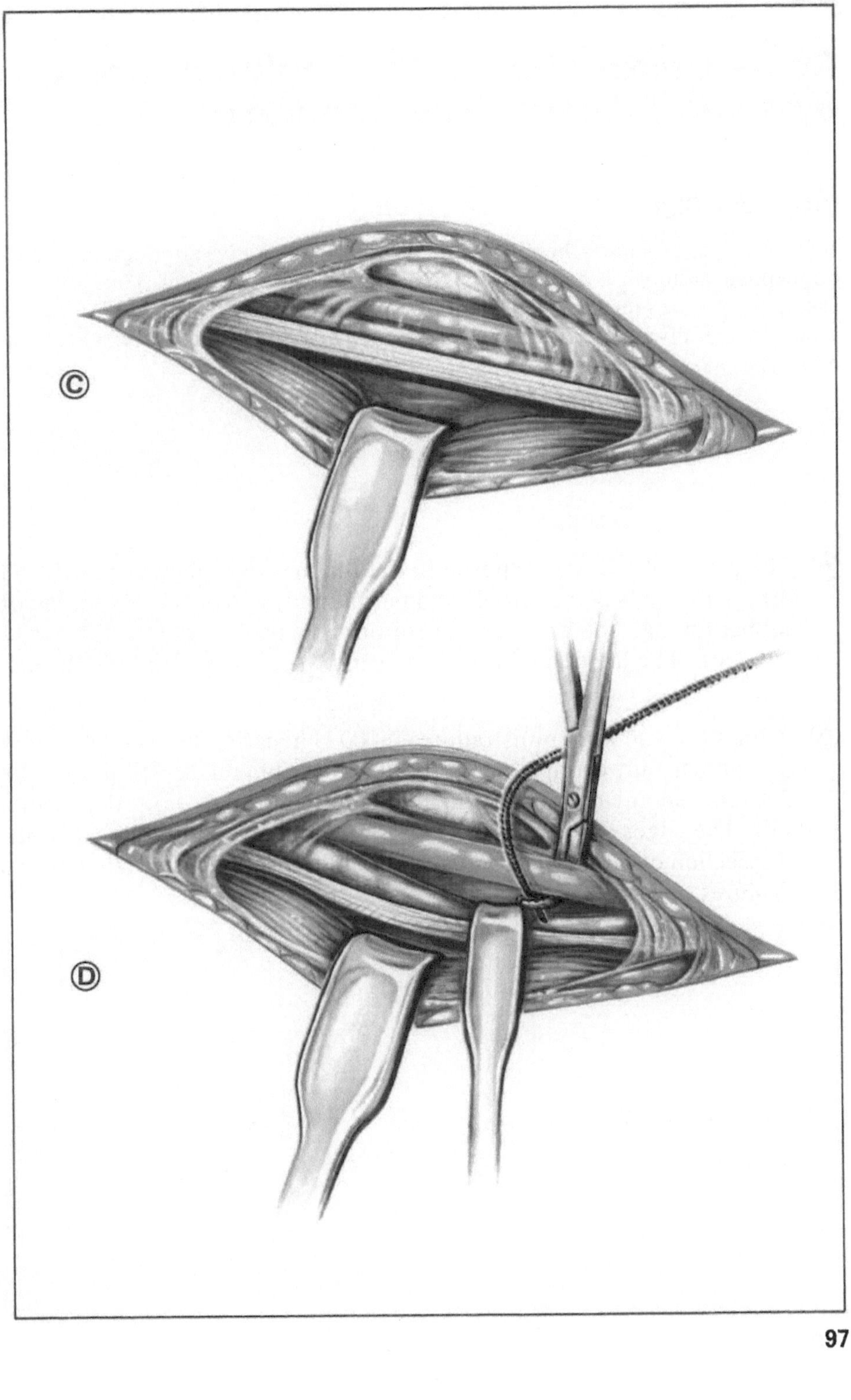
C
D

19

Acute Obstruction of the Popliteal Artery by a Thrombosed True Aneurysm

Diagnostic Signs

There are signs of acute ischemia of the lower leg. Preoperative arteriography is recommended, although it does not invariably disclose an aneurysm. Thus, in some cases, we must be prepared for a surprise finding. It is recommended to inspect the other leg carefully as well. In many cases, aneurysms of the popliteal artery are bilateral.

Ⓐ The popliteal artery is exposed in the manner described under 18 and the aneurysm is tied centrally and peripherally with thick silk thread or rubber tubing. The gastrocnemius muscle is held away in a downward direction. The large saphenous vein can be seen on the right in the picture.

Ⓑ After intravenous administration of 5000 U heparin, the popliteal artery is atraumatically clamped in a central and peripheral direction from the thrombosed aneurysm and the aneurysm is resected from the central side. The edges of the popliteal artery are marked with holding threads. If resection of the aneurysm is not possible, it is to be eliminated by two ligatures and a venous bypass is to be applied.

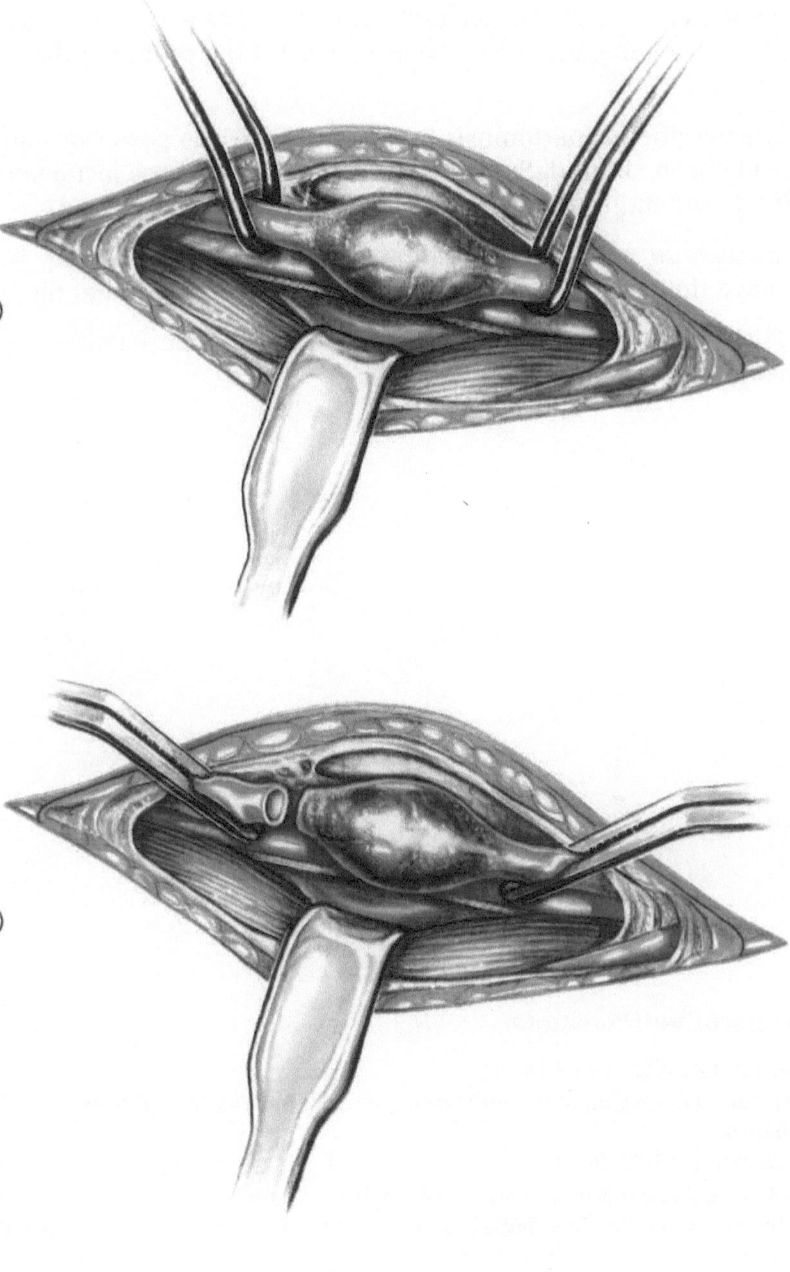

A

B

Ⓒ Status after resection of the aneurysm. A peripheral piece of the large saphenous vein is taken from the same leg. The peripheral large saphenous vein generally corresponds exactly to the caliber of the popliteal artery.

The peripheral anastomosis has been started, the posterior wall has already been sutured. Suturing of the anterior wall has just been started (with 5/0 and 6/0 monofilament double-reinforced thread).

Ⓓ Status after completed anastomosis. The atraumatic clamp is placed above the anastomosis, which can, meanwhile, close tightly.

The central anastomosis is started with the same technique and the same suturing material.

Postoperative Measures

- Redon drainage for 48 hours.
- Peripheral palpation of the pulse several times per day (possible also a control angiography).
- Antibiotic shield for 2–3 days with 2 x 2.0 g or 4 x 1.0 g Cefamandole per day.
- Anticoagulant treatment with 3 to 4 x 5000 U depot heparin per day administered subcutaneously for 3–4 days, continued with dicumarol derivative for at least 6 months.
- Mobilization on 2nd postoperative day.
- Histologic exmaination of the aneurysm.

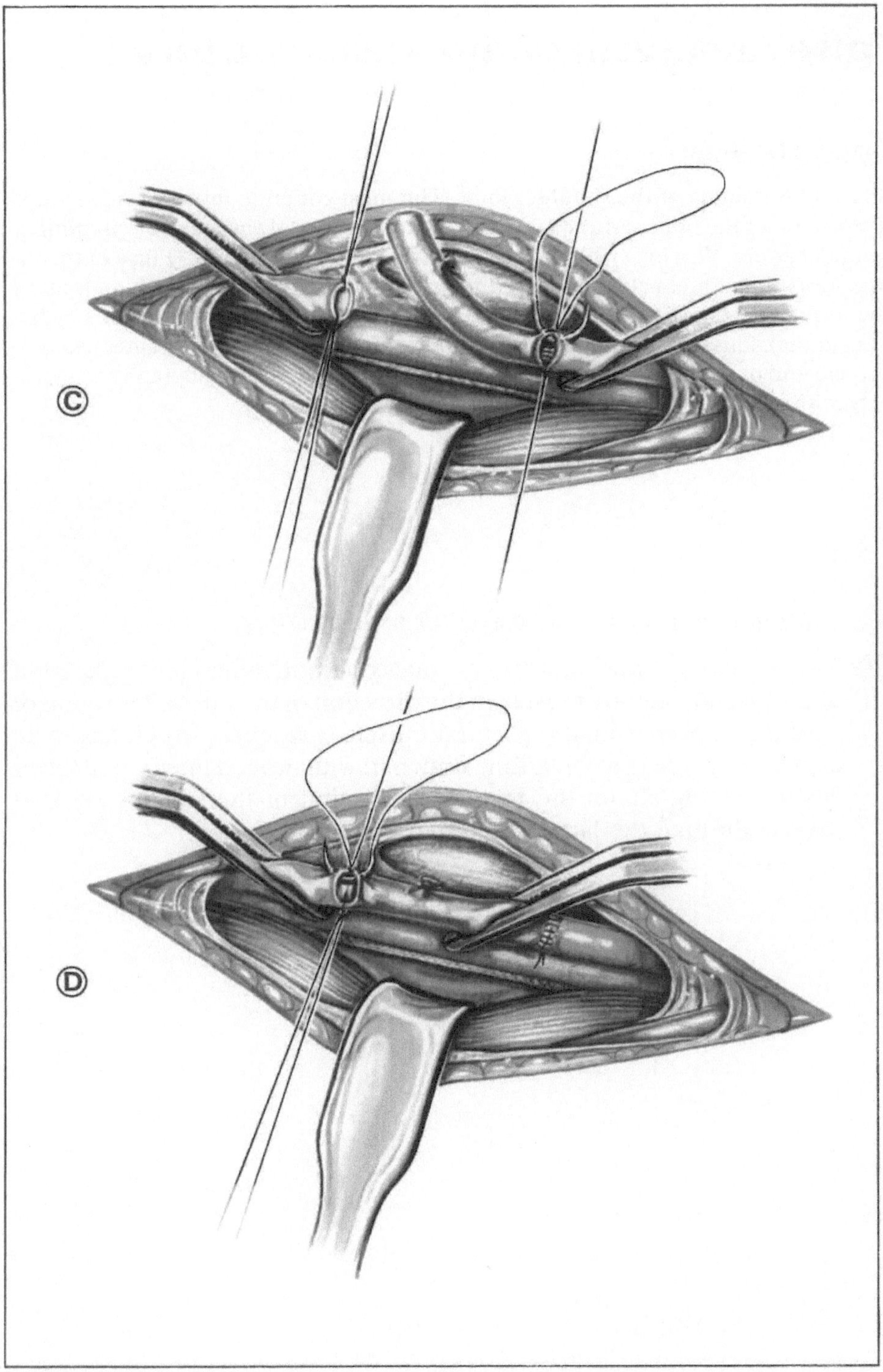
C
D

20

False Aneurysm of the Axillary Artery

Diagnostic Signs

Status after trauma of the shoulder joint. The most common injury of this kind is dislocation of the upper arm, which leads to tearing out of the anterior circumflex humeral artery. Varying symptoms of ischemia in the arm region. (Pulse of the radial artery sometimes palpable, sometimes not). Increasing neurologic symptoms in the form of paresis of the plexus (due to compression of the brachial plexus by the hematoma). Pulsating tumor in the area of the lateral portion of the greater pectoral muscle and over the shoulder joint. A transfemoral catheter angiography is necessary with selective visualization of the subclavian artery.

Ⓐ Incision to expose the subclavial or axillary artery.

Ⓑ The top smaller drawing shows normal conditions after blunt separation of the greater pectoral muscle in the direction of the fibers. The point of attachment of the smaller pectoral muscle is reached, which has to be cut transversally (line of cutting drawn in with broken lines). The lower larger drawing shows the forward projection of the smaller pectoral muscle through the large pulsating hematoma.

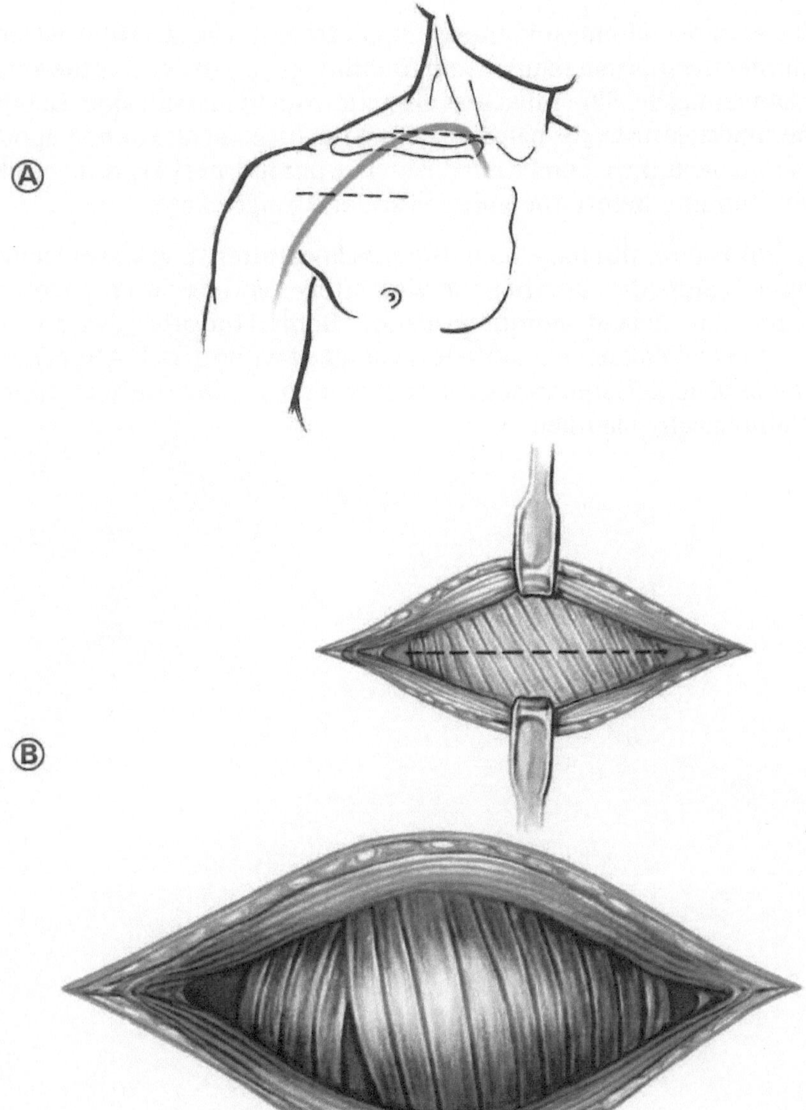

Ⓒ As shown by drawing A, an incision is made over the sternoclavicular joint. The clavicular portion of the sternocleidomastoid muscle is cut.

Ⓓ The sternocleidomastoid muscle is cut from the lateral side and we encounter the internal jugular vein. Behind the jugular vein is the anterior scalene muscle. The muscle is also cut from the lateral side. Behind it, the subclavial artery is palpable before the brachial plexus and upon further preparation, it comes into view. The phrenic nerve should be observed, running before the anterior scalene muscle and

Ⓔ is held aside with a loop. Now, the subclavial artery is readily reached an in this region, the superficial cervical artery may be injured. In this case, it should be ligated without hesitation. Behind the artery, we recognize the brachial plexus. It should be kept intact without fail. After administration of 5000 U depot-heparin (intravenously), the subclavial artery is atraumatically clamped.

Ⓒ

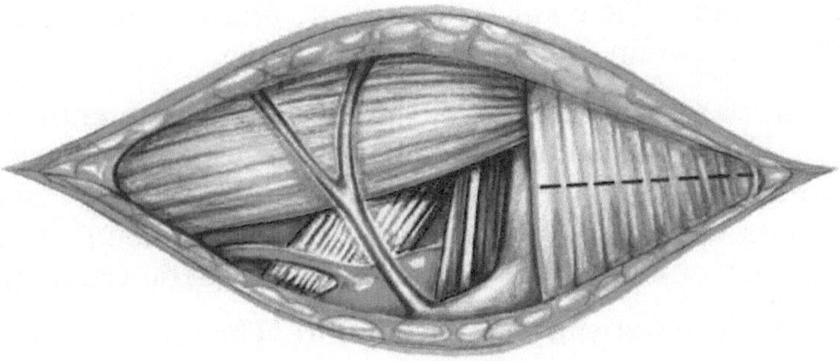

Ⓓ

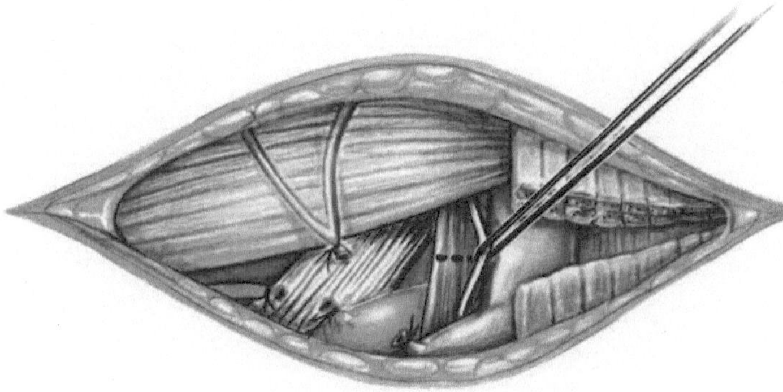

Ⓔ

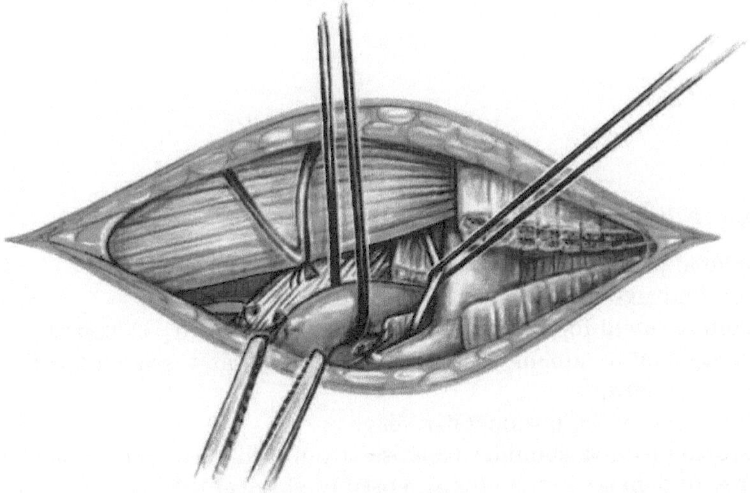

Ⓕ Normally after oblique cutting of the smaller pectoral muscle, we reach the axillary artery directly, whose preparation is very simple from this point of access. The cranial fibers of the brachial plexus must sometimes be held to one side by means of a loop.

Ⓖ This shows a typical picture of the tearing out of the anterior circumflex humeral artery in luxation of the shoulder. Despite central clamping of the subclavial artery, there is still fairly severe bleeding from the tear site (reflux bleeding). The bleeding is stopped by compression with a sponge-stick or controlled by atraumatic peripheral clamping.

Ⓗ The defect is closed with a simple U suture. The peripheral stump of the anterior circumflex humeral artery is ligated.

The hematoma is carefully cleaned out to prevent infection.

Postoperative Measures

- Peripheral palpation of the pulse several times per day.
- Redon drainage for 48 hours.
- Antibiotic shield for 2-3 days with 2 x 2.0 g or 4 x 1.0 g Cefamandole per day.
- Anticoagulant treatment, may be necessary only as possible prevention of pulmonary embolisms.
- Mobilization on 1st postoperative day.
- Active and passive shoulder exercises from 10th postoperative day.
- In case of damage to the plexus, possibly physical therapy.

Ⓕ

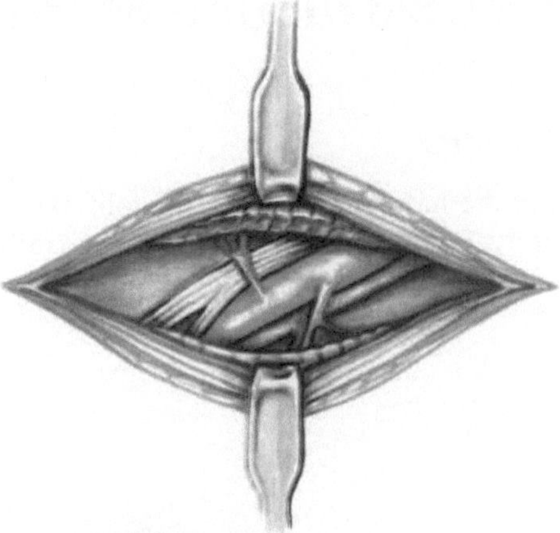

Ⓖ

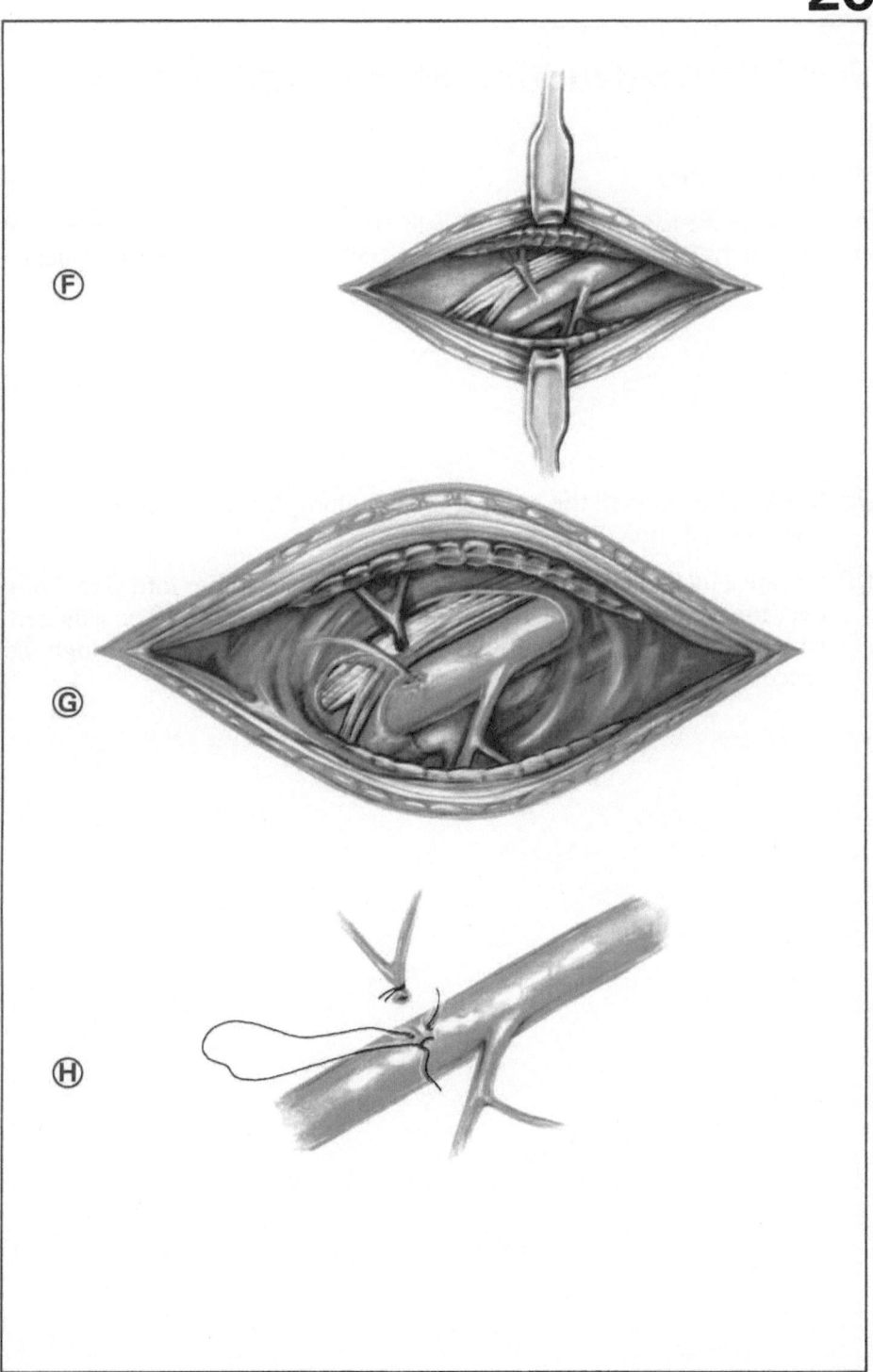

Ⓗ

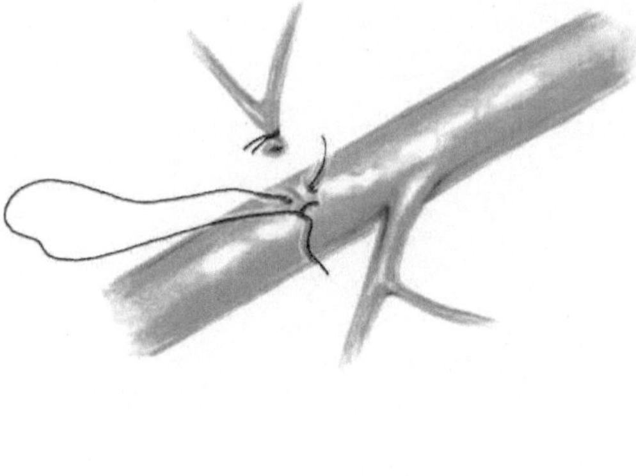

21

Embolic Obstruction of the Cubital Artery

Diagnostic Signs

Acute pain in the hand and lower arm, cold extremity, pulselessness of the radial and ulnar artery. Study of case history for signs (mitral valve defect, atrial fibrillation or the like).

Ⓐ S-shaped incision in the bend of the left elbow from an upper medial to lower lateral direction.

Ⓑ S-shaped incision has been made, the basilic vein comes into view, lying over the lacertus fibrosus. Behind it, the cubital artery can be palpated, which is displaced at this point by the embolus that shines through the vascular wall.

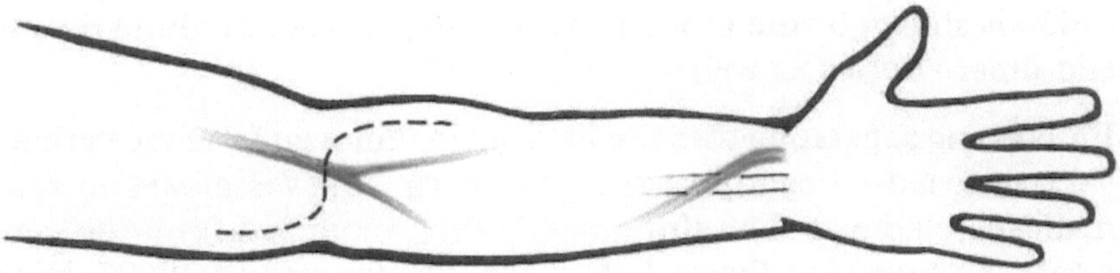

Ⓐ

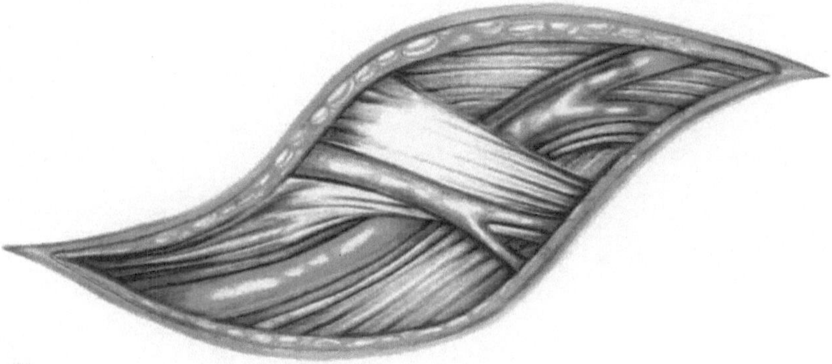

Ⓑ

21

Ⓒ The lacertus fibrosus is cut. The basilic vein has been ligated and cut. The cubital artery is exposed just above its bifurcation into radial and ulnar artery and tied. The blackishbrown embolus can be seen through the wall of the vessel. No pulse can now be palpated beneath the embolic obstruction. The site of the oblique arteriotomy just above the bifurcation is shown by the broken line. Loops are placed around the radial and ulnar arteries as well.

Ⓓ Emboli and separating thrombi have been removed from the peripheral side with a No. 4 Fogarty catheter. The peripheral vessels are now atraumatically clamped. The thrombus is then extracted from the central side with a Fogarty catheter. Before applying the clamps, 5000 U heparin was administered intravenously.

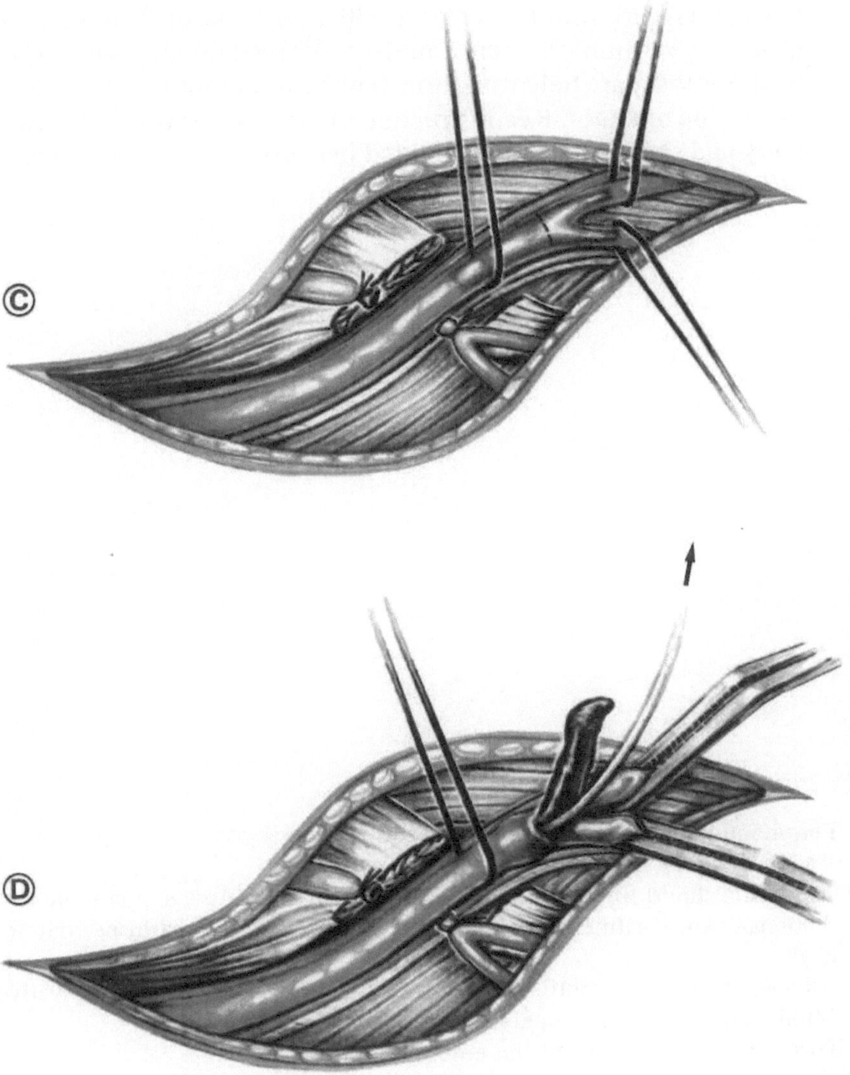
C
D

Ⓔ The embolus has been completely removed. Reflux and inflow are checked. The arteriotomy is closed with a continuous atraumatic vascular suture (6/0 monofilament double-reinforced thread). The corners of the arteriotomy are held with threads and the continuous suture is made towards the operator. Reconstruction of the lacertus fibrosus is not necessary and should indeed be omitted because of the danger of vascular compression.

Postoperative Measures

- Peripheral palpation of the pulse several times per day.
- Redon drainage for 48 hours.
- Antibiotic shield for 2–3 days with 2 x 2.0 g or 4 x 1.0 g Cefamandole per day.
- Anticoagulant treatment, with 3 to 4 x 5000 U depot heparin per day for 3–4 days.
- Change to long-term anticoagulant treatment with a dicumarol derivative.
- Mobilization on 1st postoperative day.
- Histologic examination of the embolus.

A search is made for the source of the embolism (atrial fibrillation, mitral defect, aneurysm of the subclavial artery or the like) and possibly the source of the embolism is eliminated by later surgical measures.

During the postoperative phase, a strongly bent elbow joint should be avoided. The arm should always be kept slightly stretched since a recurrent obstruction is possible in case of embolic occlusion of the cubital artery. However, a forced stretched position with a plaster splint is not advantageous.

Ⓔ

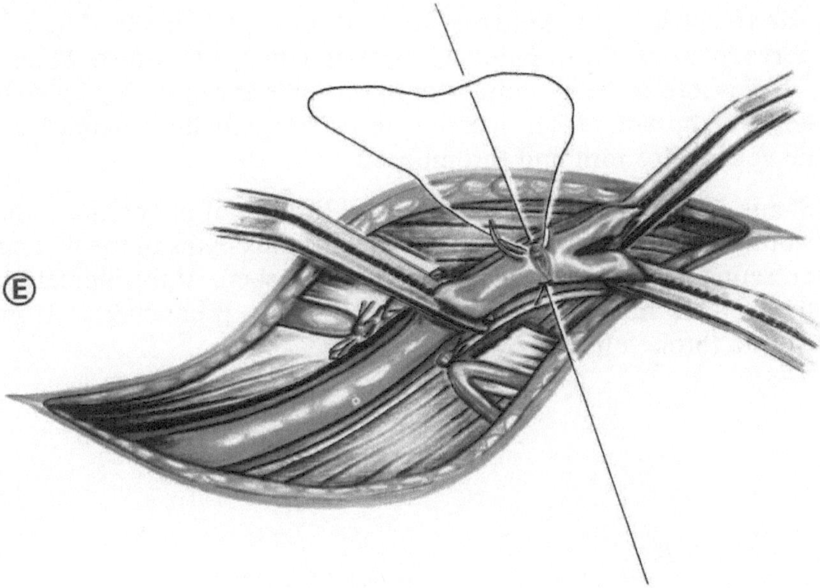

22

Open Luxation of the Lower Arm with Tearing Out of the Cubital Artery

Ⓐ Typical dorsal dislocation of the lower arm with open wound in the angle of the elbow. We are viewing the dislocated right elbow joint from the ventral side. Thus in the picture, it is left lateral and right medial. The trochlea of the humerus shows through the wound. The median nerve runs over the trochlea, it is overstretched but not torn. The cubital artery is torn out, the central stump is visible as a pulsating bulge in the depth of the wound. The lacertus fibrosus is partially torn out. The basilic vein is also torn and thrombosed.

Ⓑ Status after reposition of luxation and ligature of the basilic vein. The wound has, meanwhile, been excised. In the depths of the wound, the pulsating stump of the cubital artery can be seen. At the medial edge of the wound, the incision is extended caudally, producing an L-shaped wound (broken line).

Ⓐ

Ⓑ

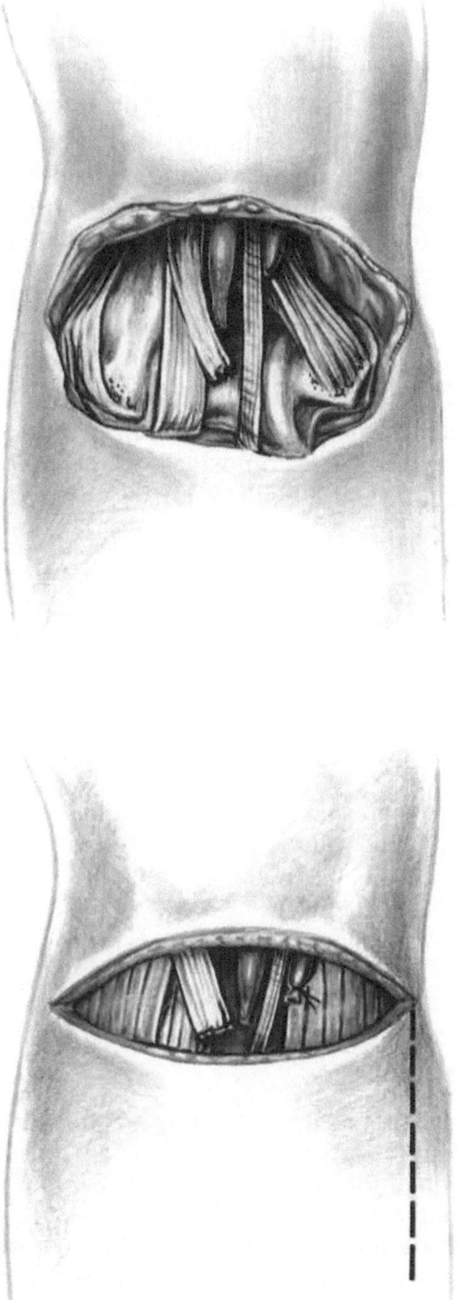

Ⓒ After extension of the wound, the peripheral portion of the cubital artery just above its bifurcation into radial and ulnar arteries is sought out. The peripheral stump is often retracted far into the muscle tissue and must be carefully prepared and sought for. It is resected far back in the healthy portion. The edges of the vessel are kept retracted by means of holding threads. The ulnar and radial arteries are atraumatically clamped and sometimes prior palpation with a Fogarty catheter and removal of separating thrombus is necessary. The atraumatic clamps are not drawn in in this picture.

Ⓓ A piece of vein from the large saphenous vein is removed from the peripheral end of the lower leg and a peripheral anastomosis is made with a 5/0 or 6/0 continuous monofilament vascular suture. The central stump of the cubital artery is resected until a completely healthy vascular wall is found. The central anastomosis is then made between the large saphenous vein and cubital artery in the manner described above.

Postoperative Measures

- Antibiotic shield with 3 x 2.0 g or 6 x 1.0 g Cefamandole per day.
- Redon drainage for 48 hours.
- Peripheral palpation of the pulse several times per day.
- Anticoagulant treatment with 3 to 4 x 5000 U depot-heparin per day subcutaneously for 4–5 days. It is not necessary to continue the anticoagulant treatment.
- Support with a Volkmann's padded upper arm splint (no plaster cast).
- Immediate mobilization.
- Active moving exercises of the elbow joint after healing of the dislocation injury.

Ⓒ

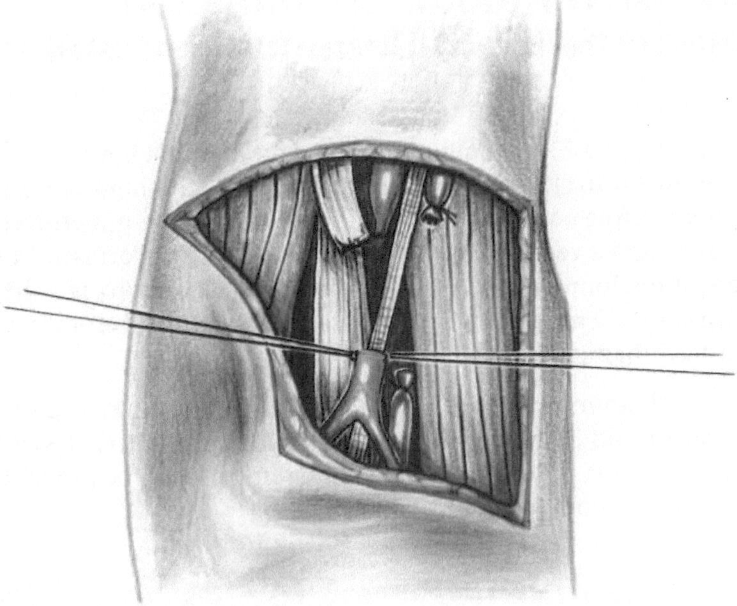

Ⓓ

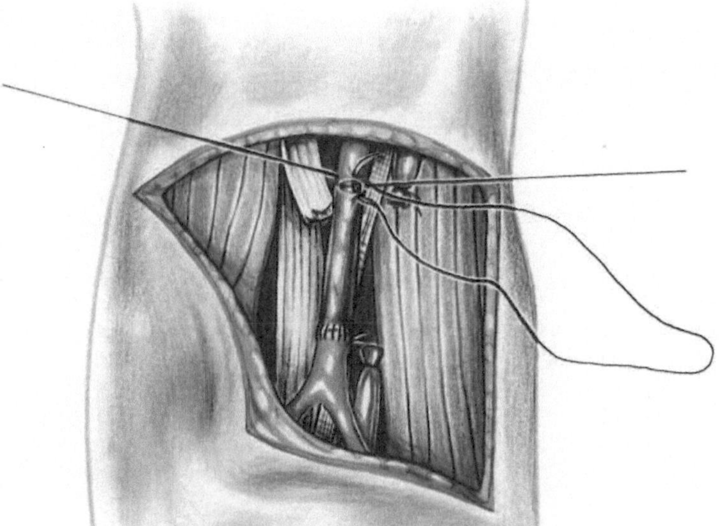

23

Operation for Inguinal Hernia with Injury to the Right Common Femoral Vein

Ⓐ Site of a typical Bassini operation for right inguinal hernia. The internal abdominal muscle was previously attached to the inguinal ligament by means of three sutures. With the fourth suture, the puncture was made too deep and a vessel was injured. At the top, the spermatic cord can be seen with a loop around it and the external aponeurosis is held with a sharp clamp. There is severe venous bleeding (the femoral artery could also have been injured).

Ⓑ With such an injury to a vein, a T-shaped extension of the herniotomy wound should be made without fail, caudally and perpendicular to the edge of the incision. Only thus can the femoral vein be prepared distally even under the inguinal ligament.

Ⓐ

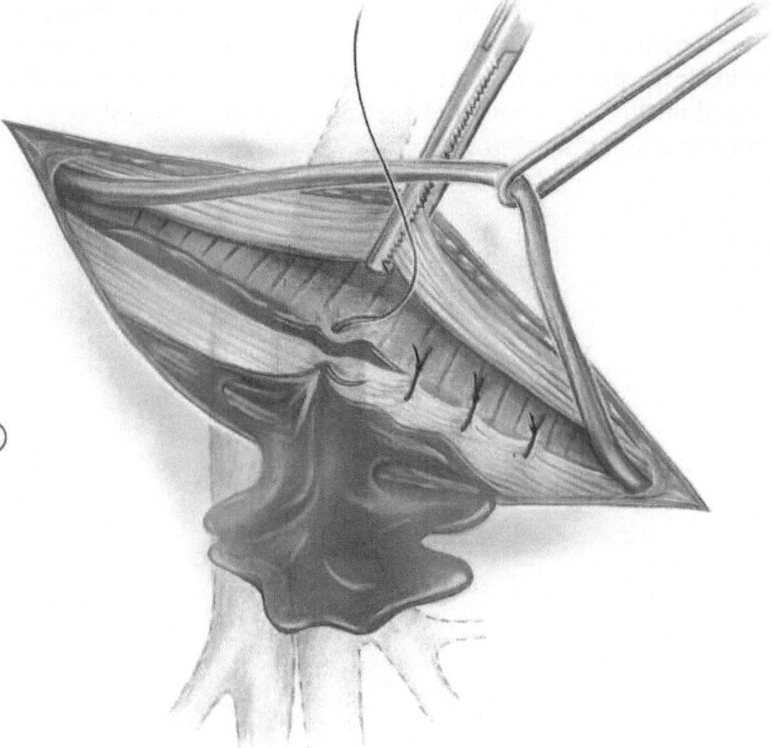

Ⓑ

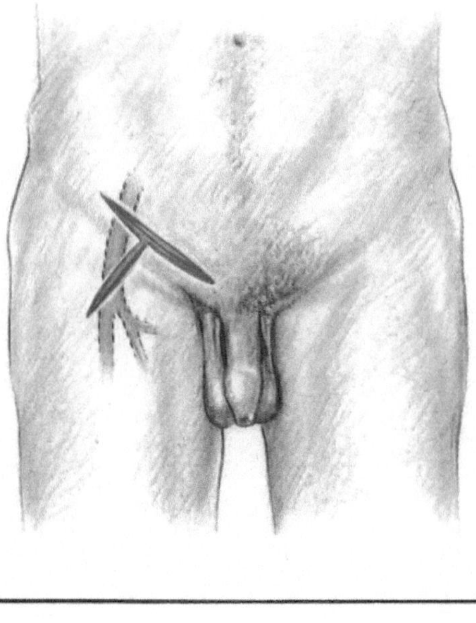

23

© After the T-shaped incision, the femoral artery and vein are prepared under the inguinal ligament. After raising the inguinal ligament, the suture can be seen with which the femoral vein was injured. At this point, the wall of the vein is sewn to the inguinal ligament. Bleeding may be severe or it may have stopped.

©

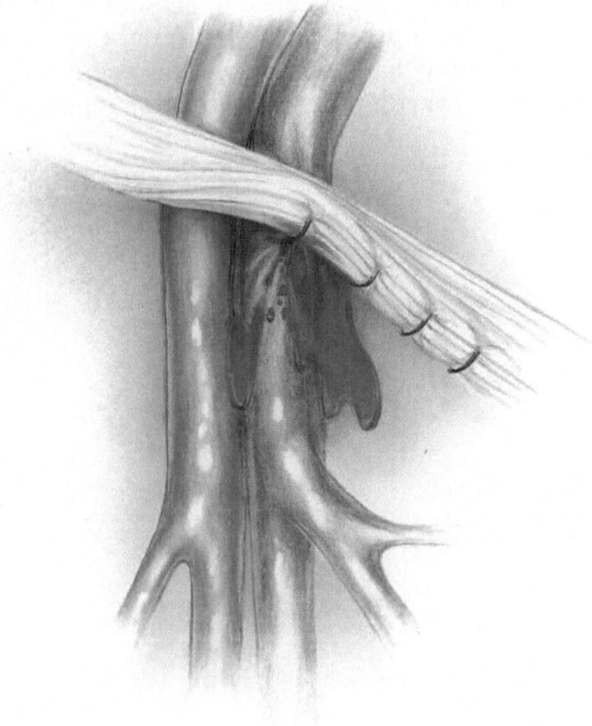

Ⓓ After sectioning the inguinal ligament from below, a good view is obtained into the site of the injury. A loop is placed distally over the femoral vein and it is compressed cranially with a sponge-stick. As a result of narrowing of the circulatory flow and injury to the vascular wall, there is almost always parietal thrombosis. Therefore, the vein must be opened in this area and the thrombus must be removed.

Ⓔ After control of bleeding by compression with a sponge-stick (not shown in picture), an oblique phlebotomy is performed in the area of the injury and the thrombus attached to the wall is removed with dressing forceps or a Fogarty catheter (on the right in picture). To check whether the thrombus has been completely removed, the clamps are temporarily opened or compression with the sponge-stick is temporarily relaxed.

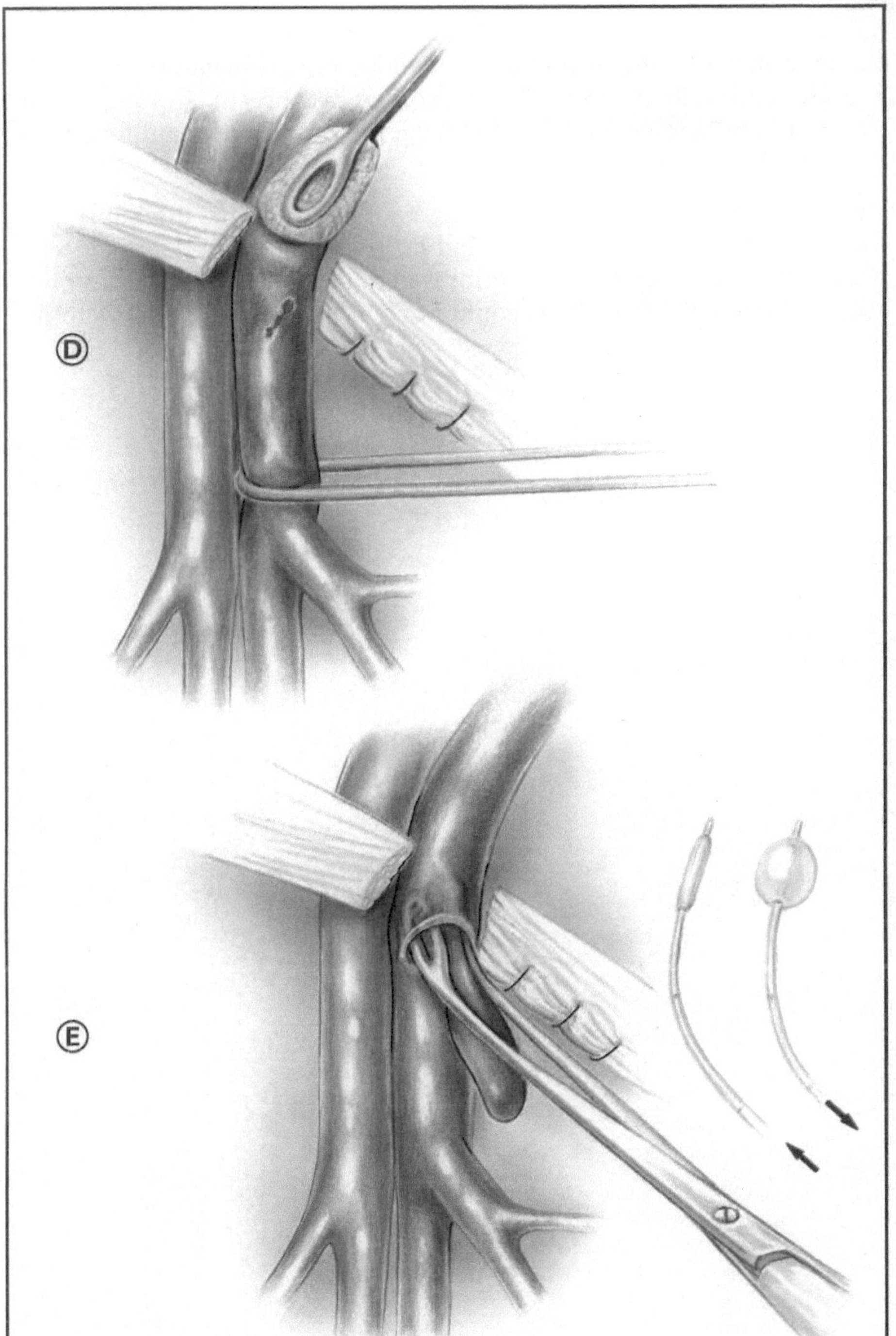
D
E

Ⓕ After removal of the thrombus, the phlebotomy is sewn up again with single interrupted sutures (5/0 monofilament thread). In the present case, the operation is completed so far as the site of venous injury is concerned.

Ⓖ It was found after sectioning the inguinal ligament that the injury was considerably more severe than had been assumed and that there was partial tearing of the entire anterior wall of the vein with total thrombosis of the femoral vein. This could not be solved with a simple suture.

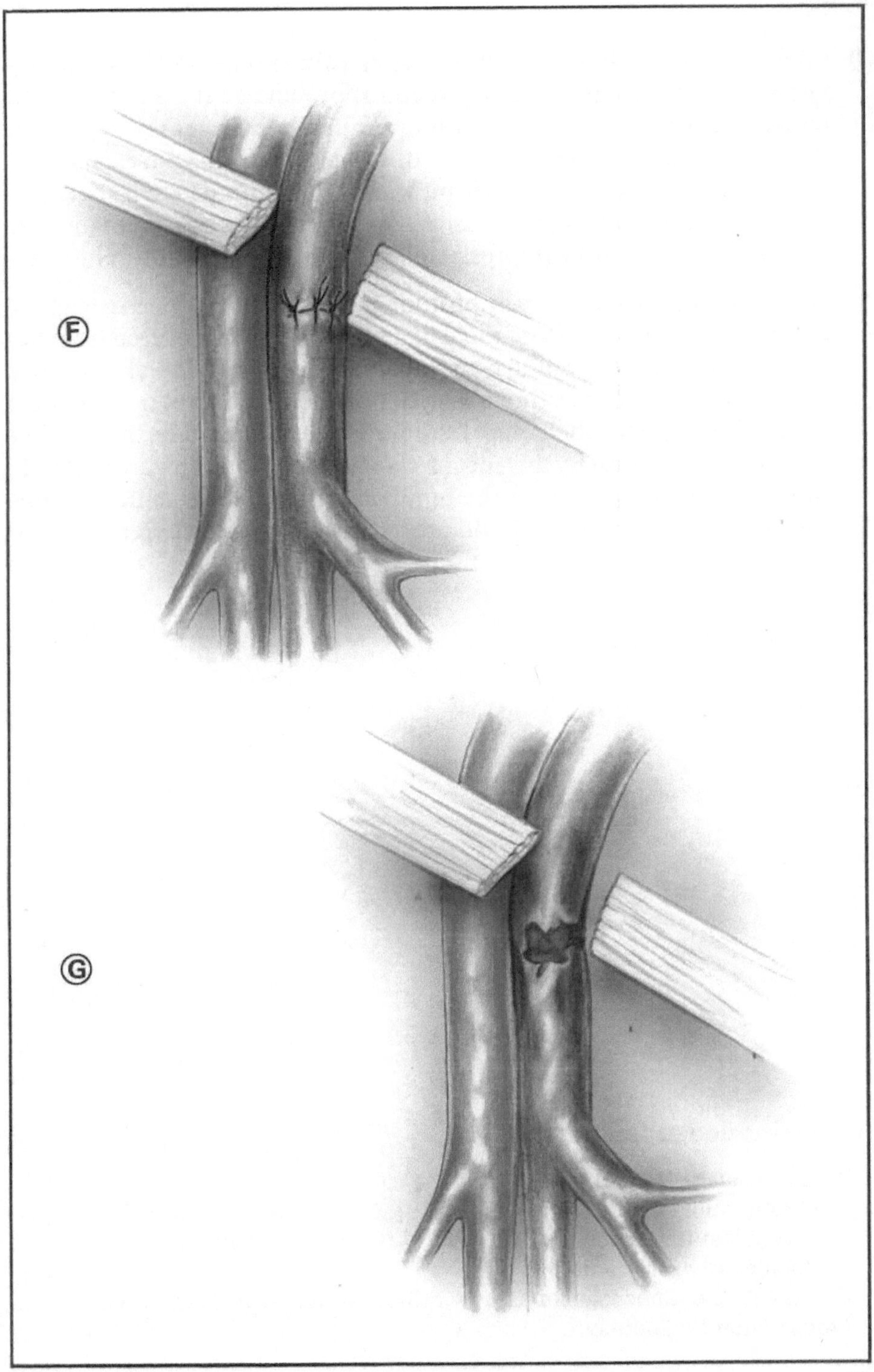
F
G

Ⓗ After resection of the injured section of vein and total thrombectomy with a Fogarty catheter from below and above and after clamping of the vessel, a plastic prosthesis (Teflon, annular reinforcement) was implanted end-to-end; a central piece of vena saphena magna can also be used if only plastic care of the front wall of the injured vein is required. In the picture, both anastomoses are completed and fastened after flushing. Clamps and compression with the swab are then removed.

Ⓘ Since a hernia operation can on longer be performed in the manner planned in the area of the inguinal ligament which was severed from below, inasmuch as this would cause inevitable compression of the newly reconstructed venous segment, a pedunculated portion of the pectineal muscle is sewn into the defect in the inguinal ligament in the manner shown in the picture. By this means, a relatively strong closure of the inguinal ligament and thus of the inguinal hernia can be achieved. Furthermore, the implanted plastic prosthesis is covered thereby.

Postoperative Measures

- Redon drainage for 48 hours.
- Antibiotic shield with 2 x 2.0 g or 4 x 1.0 g Cefamandole per day (for 3 days).
- Anticoagulant treatment, with 4 x 5000 U depot-heparin per day administered subcutaneously for 4–5 days.
- Continuation of anticoagulant treatment with Marcoumar for at least 6 months.
- Mobilization on 2nd day.

Ⓗ

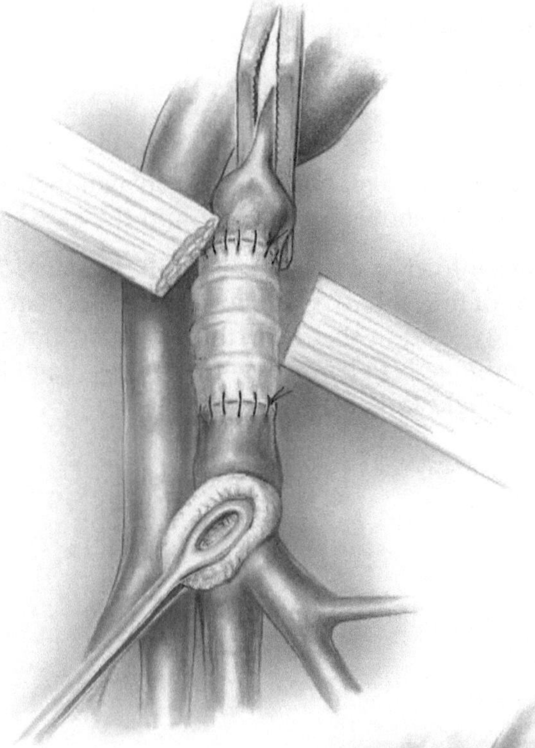

Ⓘ

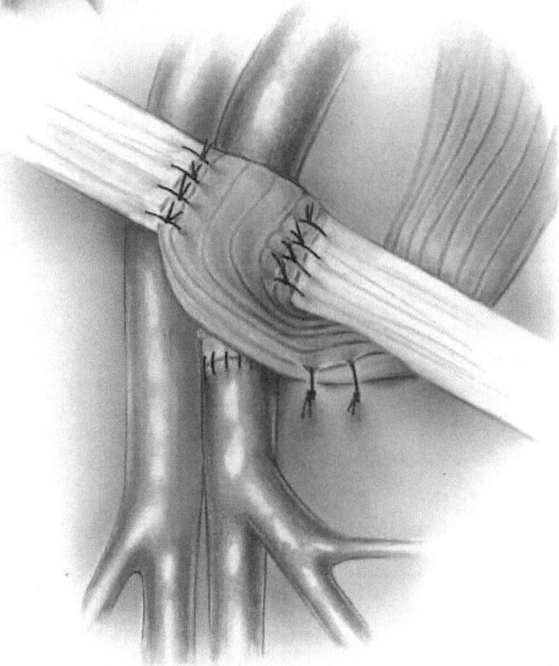

24

Injury of the Axillary Vein During Mastectomy

Ⓐ Right mammary carcinoma. The planned spindle-shaped incision over the right mammary gland is shown, extending into the axillary fossa.

Ⓑ The axillary vein comes into view while preparing the axillary fossa. As a rule, the lower border of the axillary vein should not be overstepped in a breast amputation. However, in this case, ther are suspicious lymph nodes that have to be removed. The muscular part of the caput longum of the biceps muscle is held aside.

Ⓐ

Ⓑ

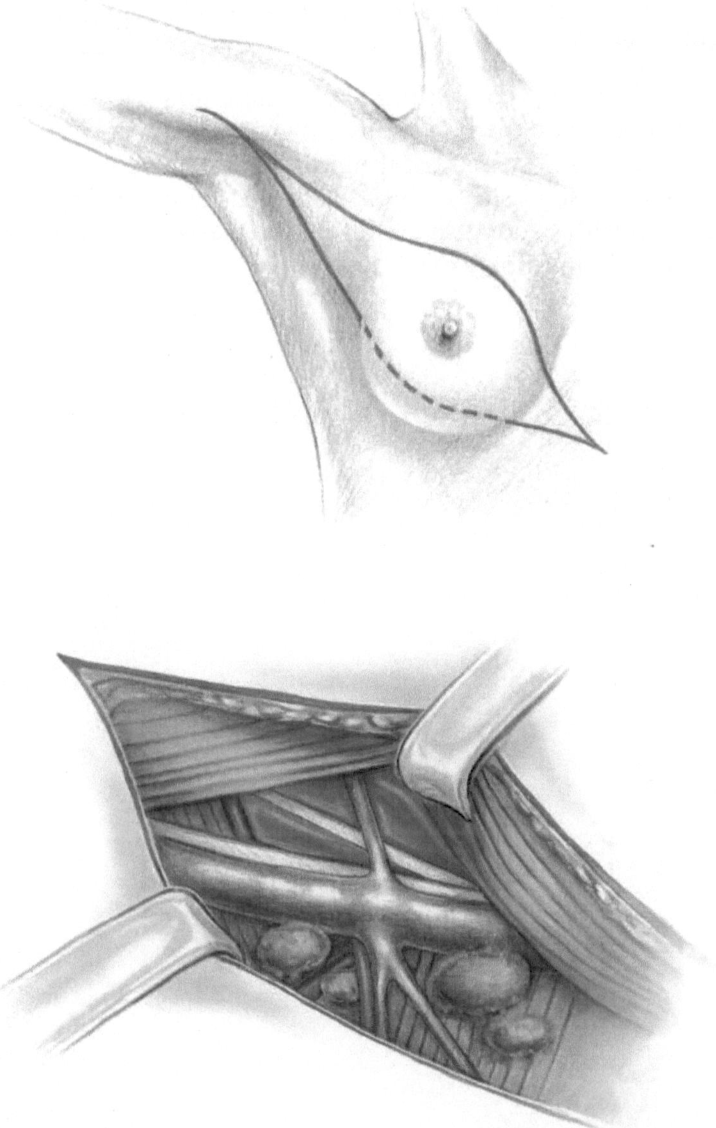

Ⓒ While preparing the macroscopically suspect lymph nodes, the axillary vein is injured with scissors. There is diffuse bleeding and it is impossible to see properly, since the field of operation is flooded. After further retraction of the muscle and compression of the efferent portion of the axillary vein,

Ⓓ the site of the injury comes into view. The blood is removed with an electric aspirator and the first suture is made, obliquely holding the site of injury. As a result of manual compression, the bleeding immediately abates. Further hemostasis can be achieved by central application of compression with a sponge-stick, although, as a rule, distal suppression of peripheral blood flow is sufficient.

Ⓒ

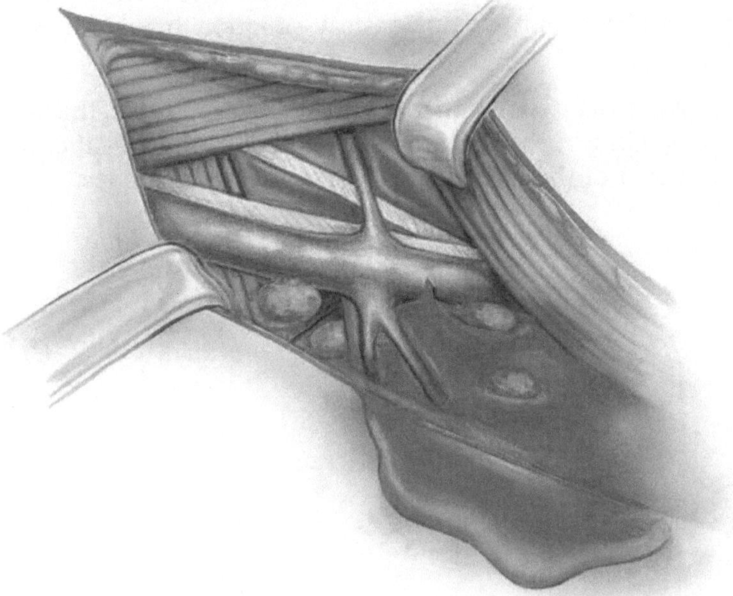

Ⓓ

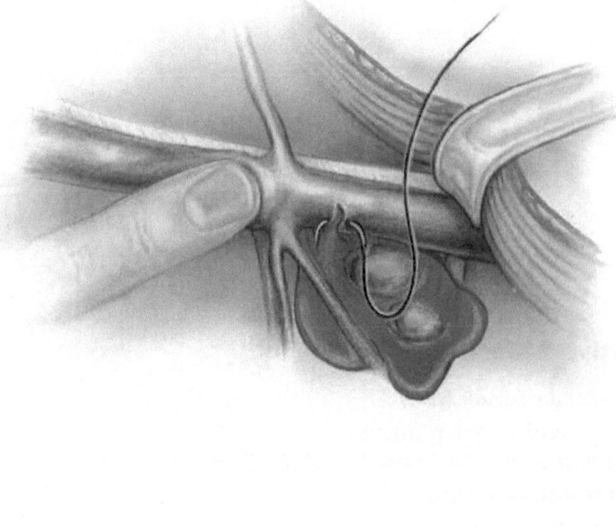

Ⓔ After continued compression and fastening of the first thread, which remains taut, a second single interrupted suture is made (5/0 monofilament thread) and the site of injury is attended to further. Bleeding continues to abate and the anatomical situation becomes recognizable again.

Ⓕ Status after final steps taken to close the site of injury of the axillary vein with single interrupted sutures and ligature of the vasa thoracolateralia and removal of the pathologically altered lymph nodes.

Postoperative Measures

- Redon drainage for 48 hours.
- Antibiotic shield is not required.
- Anticoagulant treatment with 4 x 5000 U depot-heparin for 4–5 days.
- Elevation of the right arm.
- Immediate mobilization.
- Active exercises with movement of the shoulder joint as soon as possible.
- Appropriate follow-up treatment for the carcinoma findings.

Ⓔ

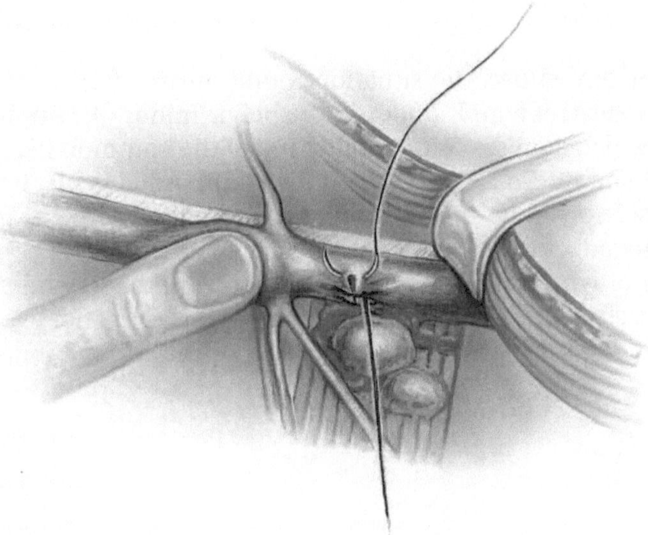

Ⓕ

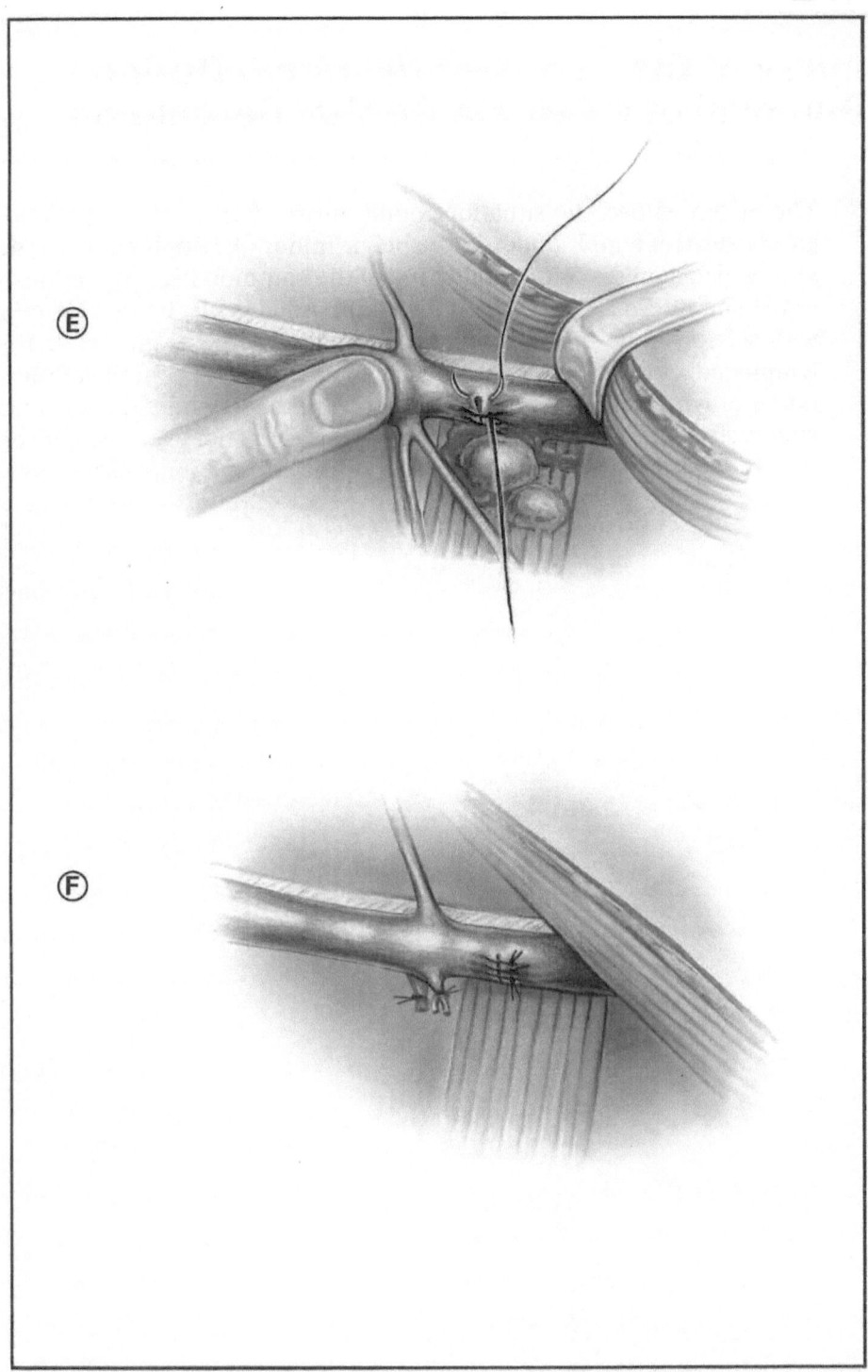

25

Injury of the Common Iliac Vein During Removal of a Female Genital Carcinoma

Ⓐ The picture shows the situation found during preparation of pathologically suspect lymph nodes in the pelvis minor. A lymph node can be seen which adheres to the branching of the common iliac vein into external and internal iliac veins. This lymph node is just being removed with scissors. The uterus is held with holding forceps and above the lymph node, the iliac artery can be seen with the ureter behind it. Preparation of lymph nodes is more dangerous in this region since the iliac vein is stretched over the pelvic bone and is often not even recognized as a vein because, due to the position of the patient, it appears empty.

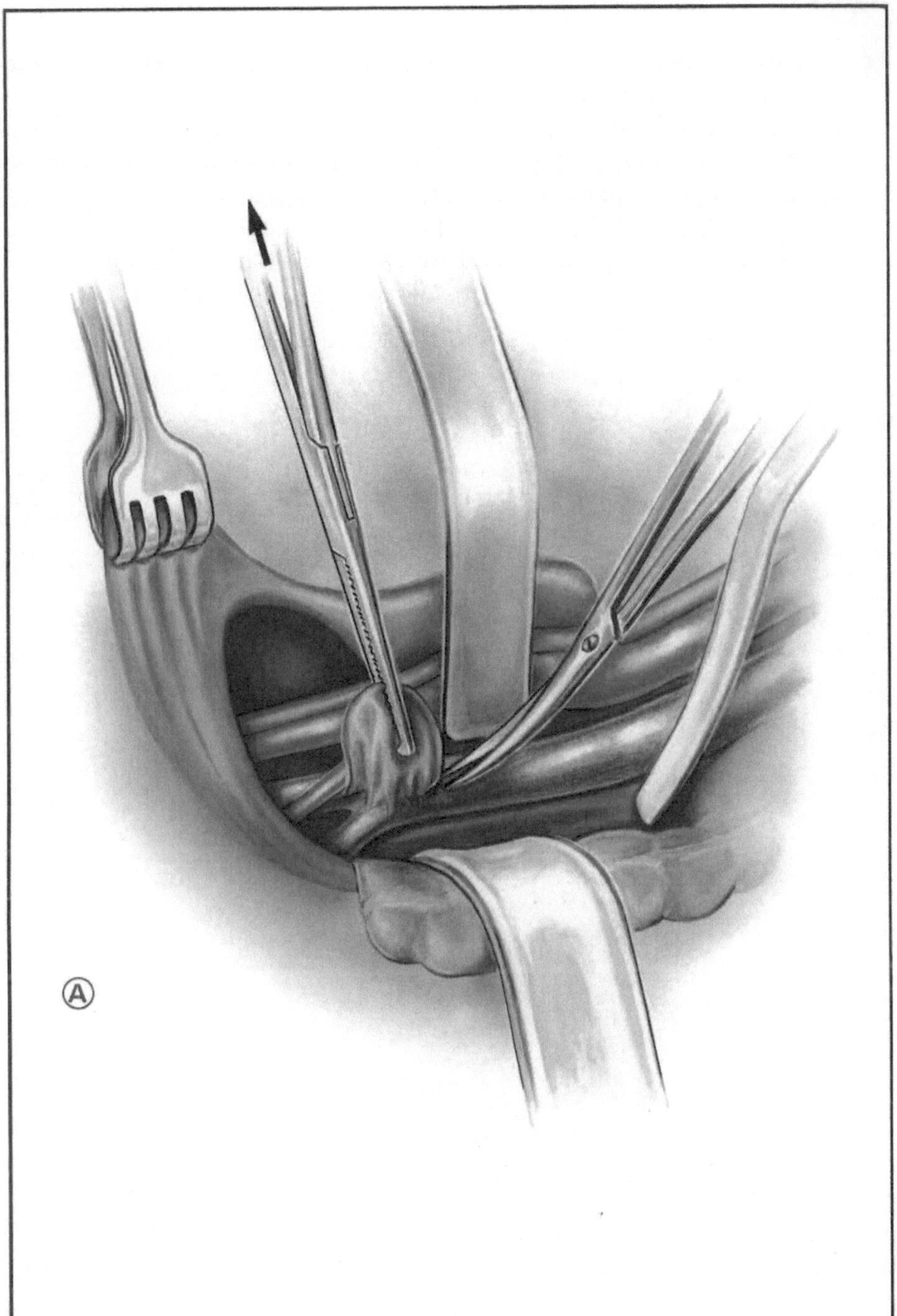

25

Ⓑ Situation after removal of the lymph node, showing injury to the anterior wall of the common iliac vein bifurcation. However, at first, the injury cannot be located because of the severe bleeding. It should be noted that venous hemorrhaging cannot be pinpointed due to rapid flooding of the field of operation, in contrast to arterial bleeding, which spurts away from the field of operation. The very first measure here is installation of a second aspirator to create clearly visible conditions.

Remark: Sharp clamps should never be used blindly, even if the situation is highly dramatic.

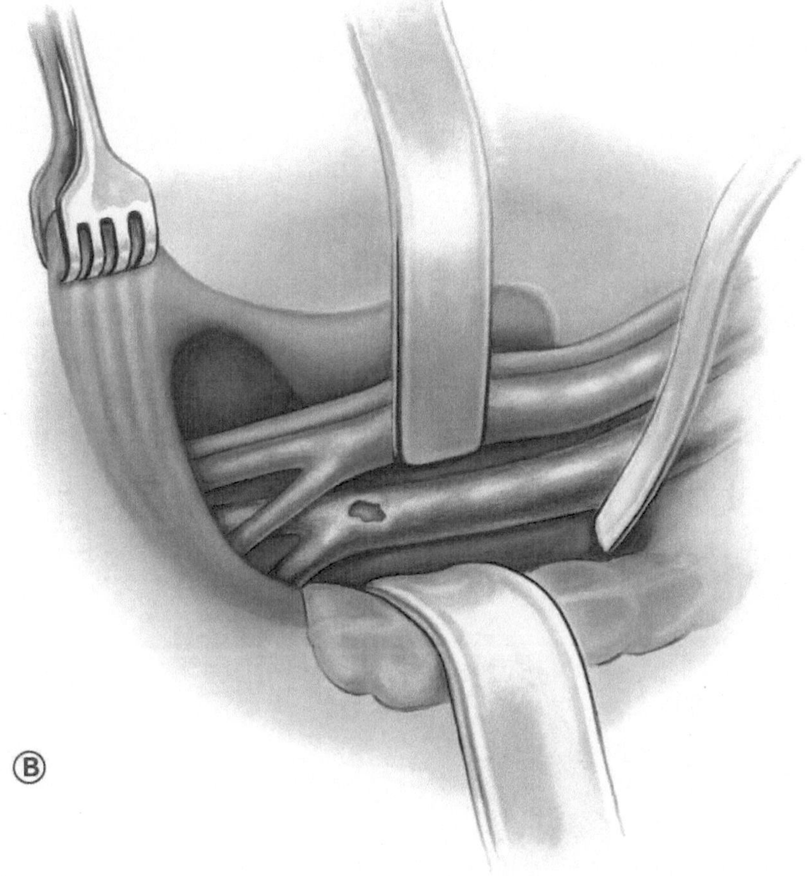
B

25

© The only possibility for bringing such a hemorrhage under control is by compression of the iliac vein with a sponge-stick above and below the site of injury. Now, the defect in the anterior wall of the vein is distinctly visible. In the picture, the first single interrupted suture is being made, with wich the injury is being closed. A loop is placed around the iliac artery and it is held aside to obtain a good view. The injured edges of the vein must be held, thus raising the anterior wall away from the posterior wall.

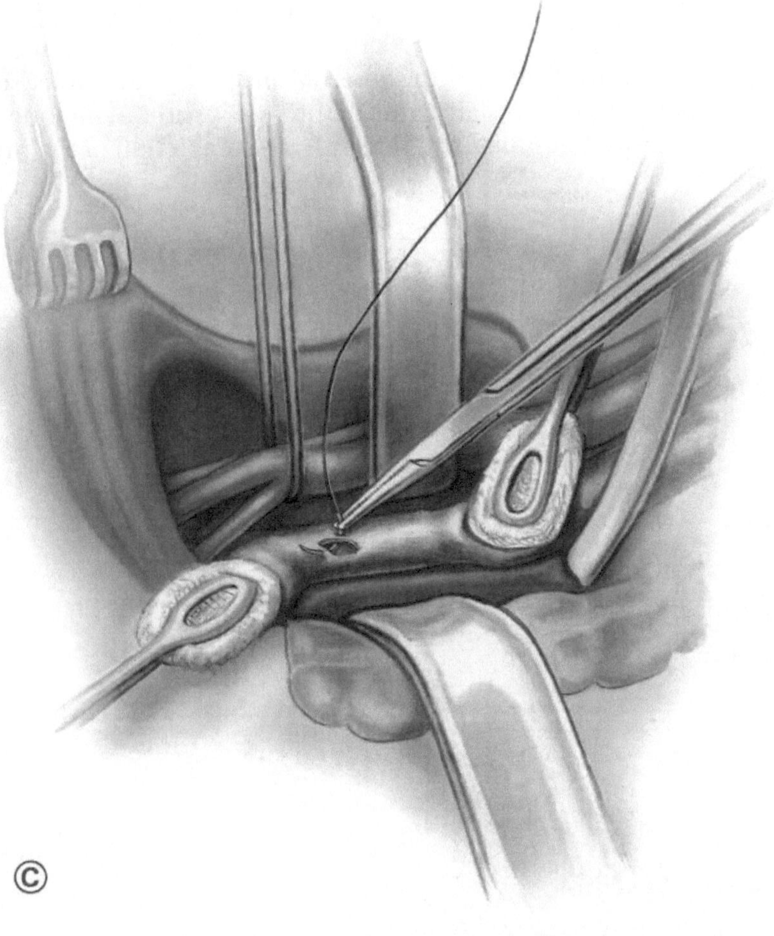

©

Ⓓ With the first suture, the site of the injury is drawn upwards to form a lip so that with the second suture, which is just being made, the anterior wall can be accurately grasped. This double suture is fastened and while holding the thread,

Ⓔ a third suture is made with which, as a rule, the injured site can be finally closed. This suture may cause some narrowing of the iliac vein, since there was previously a defect. This narrowing, indicated by the arrows, can be disregarded since the collateral blood flow functions well through the sacral plexus and the internal iliac veins and thus some degree of narrowing of the main trunk of the vein is without importance. The picture shows the situation after suturing completion of the injury site.

Postoperative Measures

- Redon drainage for 48 hours (depending on gynecologic needs).
- Antibiotic shield with 2 x 2.0 g or 4 x 1.0 g Cefamandole per day.
- Anticoagulant treatment with 4 x 5000 U depot heparin per day for 4–5 days.
- Continuation of Marcoumar treatment is recommended, based on consultation with the gynecologist.
- Compression bandage of the leg in question.
- If possible, mobilization on 2nd postoperative day.

Ⓓ

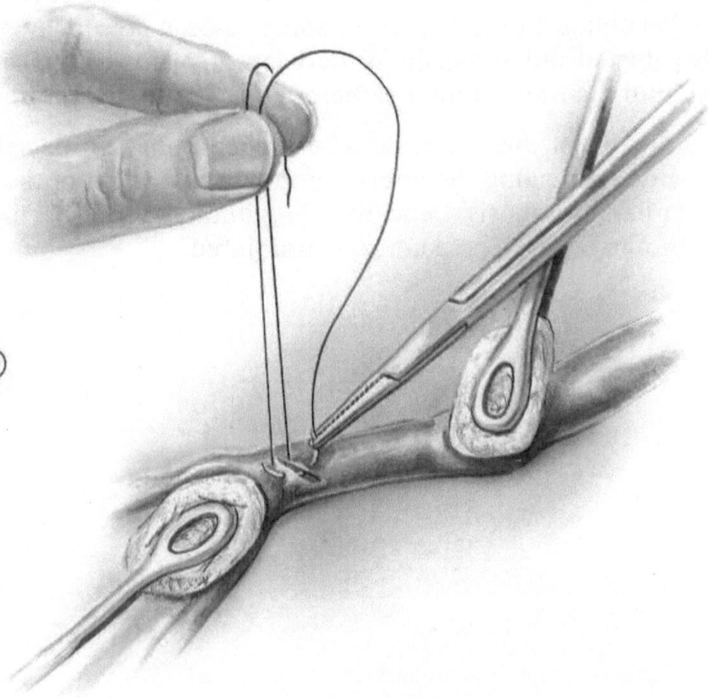

Ⓔ

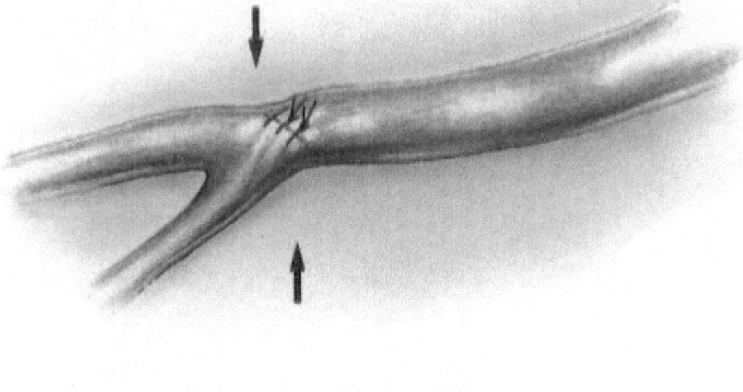

26

Closed Fracture of the Shaft of the Humerus with Injury of the Brachial Artery

Ⓐ This is a sharp oblique fracture of the humerus with impalement of the brachial artery by the distal fragment. Diagnosis: absence of peripheral pulse and symptoms of ischemia. In some cases, a pulse may be alternatingly palpated and lost again. If there is a suspicion of such a closed brachial injury, a transfemoral catheter angiography is required.

Ⓑ Detailed picture of the situation. The broken bone can be seen, the distal fragment impaling the artery. In the distal portion of the artery, there is partial thrombosis. Beneath it, longitudinally, there is a portion of median nerve in the present case, uninjured.

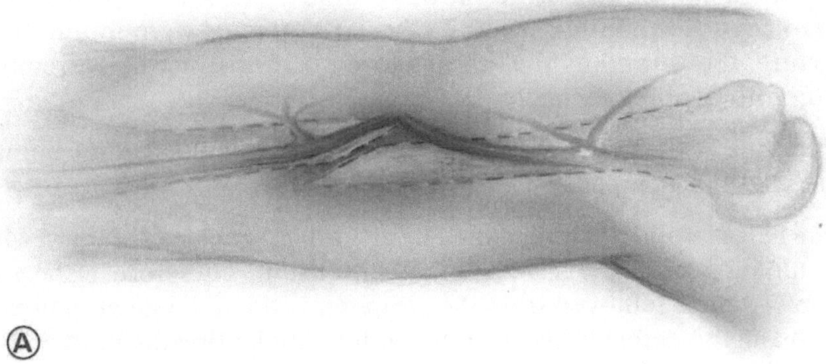

Ⓐ

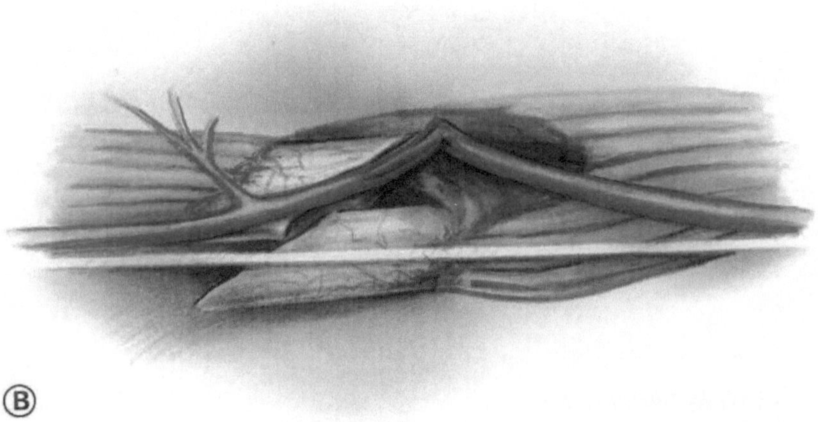

Ⓑ

Ⓒ Meanwhile, the injured humerus has been set from the lateral side with a plate osteosynthesis. The tips of the screws can be seen in the picture. The fracture fissure is still visible. The fracture is stabilized. A basic principle in caring for combined bone and vascular injuries is: first, stabilization of the bone (as quickly as possible!) and only then, vascular reconstruction. The picture shows that meanwhile, the brachial artery has been resected until healthy vascular segments were found. In the picture, the thrombus that always forms there is just being removed from the peripheral side.

The edge of the artery is held with a suture, while the central stump of the artery is clamped.

Ⓓ The defect could not be spanned by an end-to-end anastomosis, which would most probably have been under tension. Therefore, a short section of vein is removed from the peripheral end of the great saphenous vein and the defect is bridget over with it, implanting the graft end-to-end. The technique is the same as in examples previously described. Next, the blood flow is released. Bone stabilized. Vessel reconstructed.

Postoperative Measures

- Peripheral palpation of the pule several times per day.
- Redon drainage for 48 hours.
- Antibiotic shield with 2 x 2.0 g or 4 x 1.0 g Cefamandole per day.
- Anticoagulant treatment with 3 to 4 x 5000 U depot heparin per day for 3-4 days.
- Continuation of anticoagulant treatment not required.
- Immobilization according to consultation with the traumatologist, probably only briefly.
- Immediate mobilization of the patient.

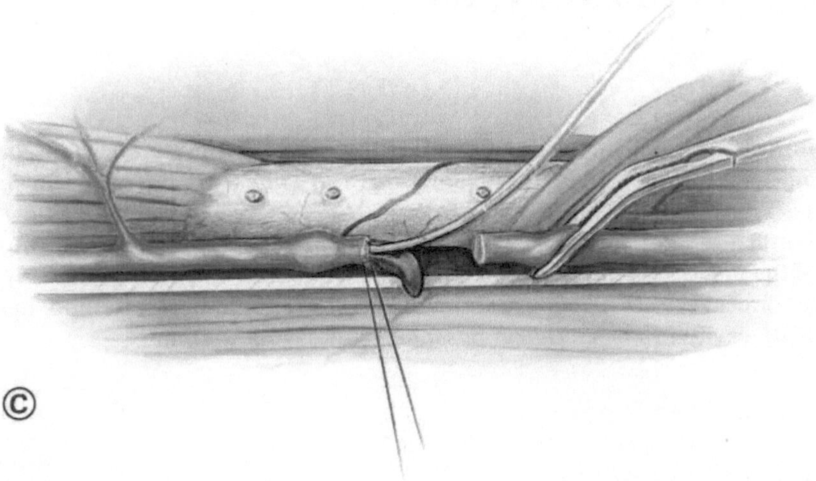

Ⓒ

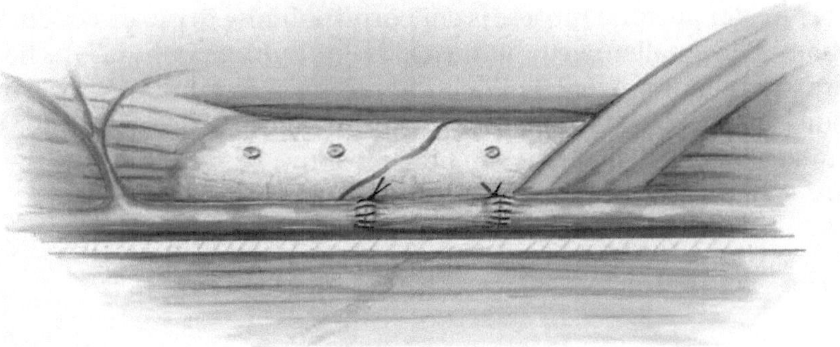

Ⓓ

27

Exposure of the Axillary Artery Distal to the Clavicle for Grafting an Emergency Axillo-femoral Bypass

Diagnostic Signs

Grafting of an emergency axillo-femoral bypass may be considered when a patient is being operated upon under the assumption of an acute embolic femoral occlusion and it is then found that despite the thrombectomy, there is still no blood flow from the central direction. Thus, there is undoubtedly an older (arteriosclerotic) obstruction of the iliac artery. If the patient's condition does not allow a (functionally preferable) direct aorto-iliac reconstruction, an axillo-femoral bypass without opening of a body cavity offers a surgical possibility for saving the limb.

Ⓐ Longitudinal incision over the peripheral portion of the greater pectoral muscle over the course of the axillary artery.

Ⓑ The greater pectoral muscle is cut corresponding to the direction of the fibers. The smaller pectoral muscle is cut through obliquely. The axillary artery is immediately encountered on a distal branch of which a loop is being placed, while a loop has already been placed over the main trunk. The brachial plexus can be seen above it and beneath it, the axillary vein.

Ⓐ

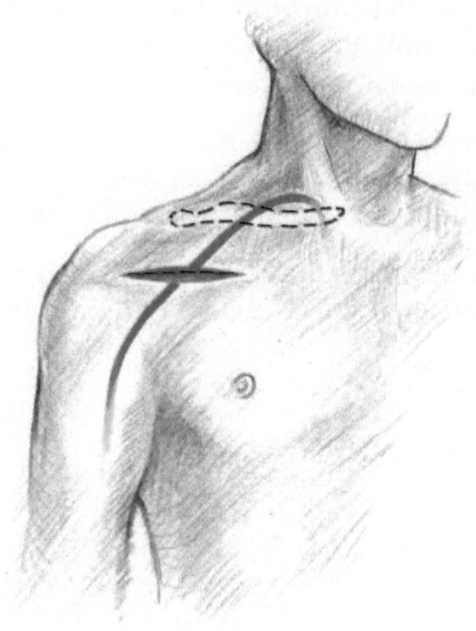

Ⓑ

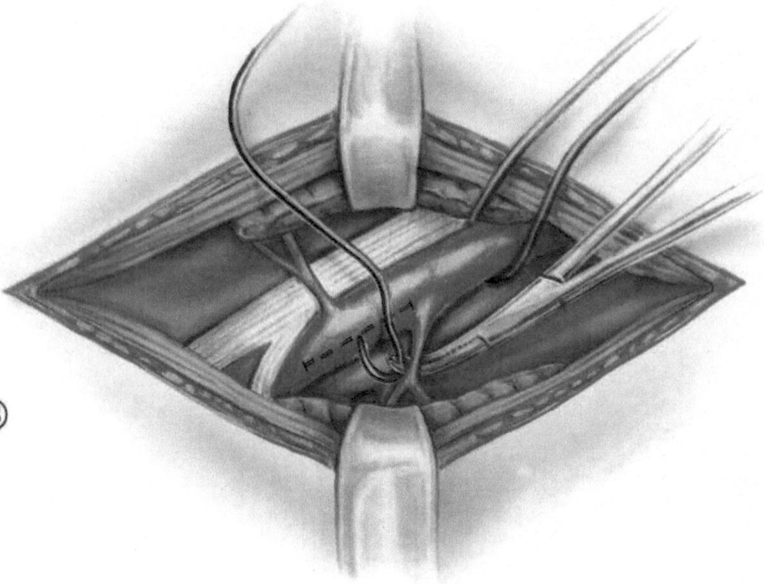

Ⓒ After clamping, the axillary artery is opened lengthwise and anastomosed obliquely side-to-end with a dacron prosthesis. If possible, the collateral vessels (at the top in picture) should be looped and only temporarily tied. The posterior wall has already been sutured and suturing of the anterior wall of the vessel is just taking place.

Ⓓ The drawings show schematically that the angle of departure of the axillo-femoral bypass should not be T-shaped (left), but oblique (right), so as to maintain the hemodynamic principles of blood distribution.

The axillo-femoral bypass is drawn subcutaneously across the medioclavicular line using an auxiliary incision on the lateral side of the thorax and chest.

Ⓒ

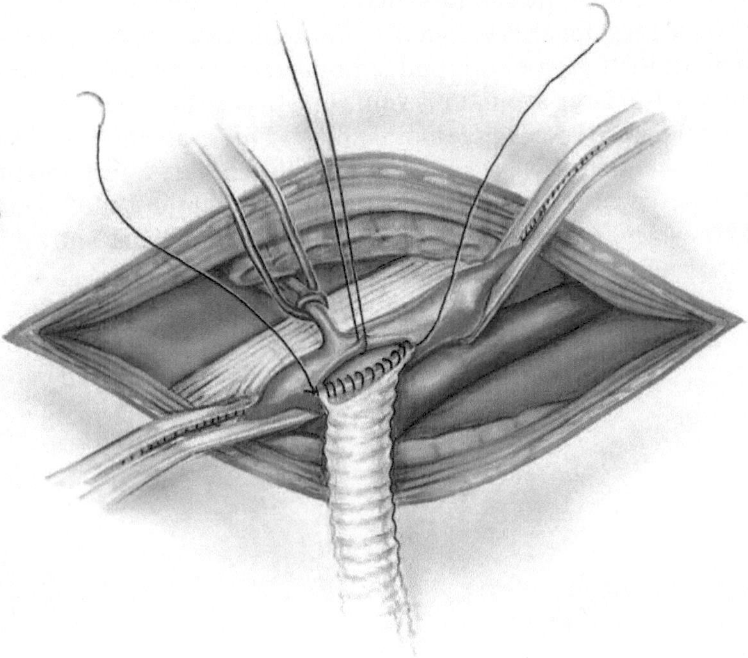

Ⓓ

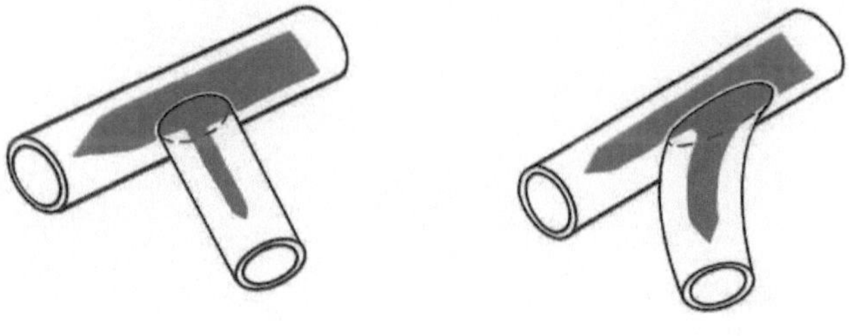

27

Ⓔ The picture shows the situation in the groin. A loop is placed around the superficial femoral artery. In most cases, this vessel is occluded. On the right in the picture, the common femoral vein can be seen with the point of entry of the large saphenous vein. The bypass has been sewn up over the initial part of the deep femoral artery. This is an end-to-side anastomosis between the bypass passing under the axillary artery and the deep femoral artery. Preparation of the deep femoral artery should continue up to the point of departure of the first main branch, as shown here in the drawing.

Postoperative Measures

- Palpation of the pulse in the area of the axillofemoral bypass several times per day.
- Redon drainage for 48 hours.
- Antibiotic screen with 2 x 2.0 g or 4 x 1.0 g Cefamandole daily for 3–5 days.
- Anticoagulant treatment with 3 to 4 x 5000 U depot heparin per day administered subcutaneously for 4–5 days.
- Continuation of anticoagulant treatment according to possibilities.
- No immobilization.
- Patient should be mobilized on 2nd postoperative day.

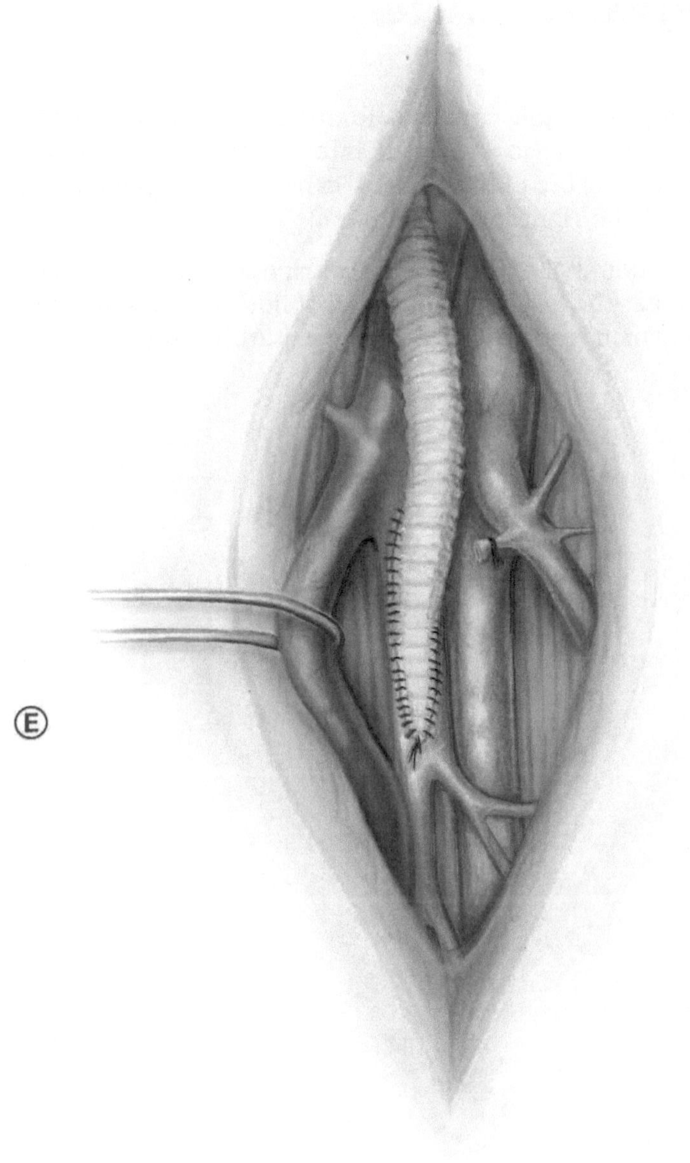

28

Emergency Exposure of Right External Iliac Artery

Ⓐ There is an injury of the common femoral artery which cannot be clamped locally (large false aneurysm, infected vascular wound). Distal retroperitoneal exposure of the vessel is carried out. A small incision is made distally in the right lower abdomen.

Ⓑ The external abdominal muscle is cut corresponding to the direction of the fibers as far as the fascia. The internal oblique abdominal muscle is encountered, which is cut obliquely in the picture, corresponding to the broken line.

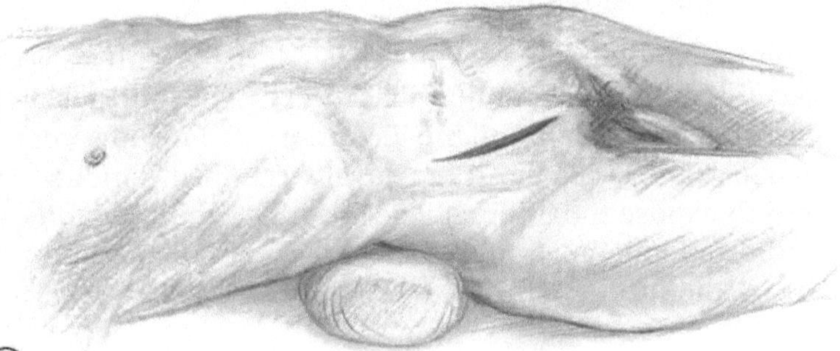

Ⓐ

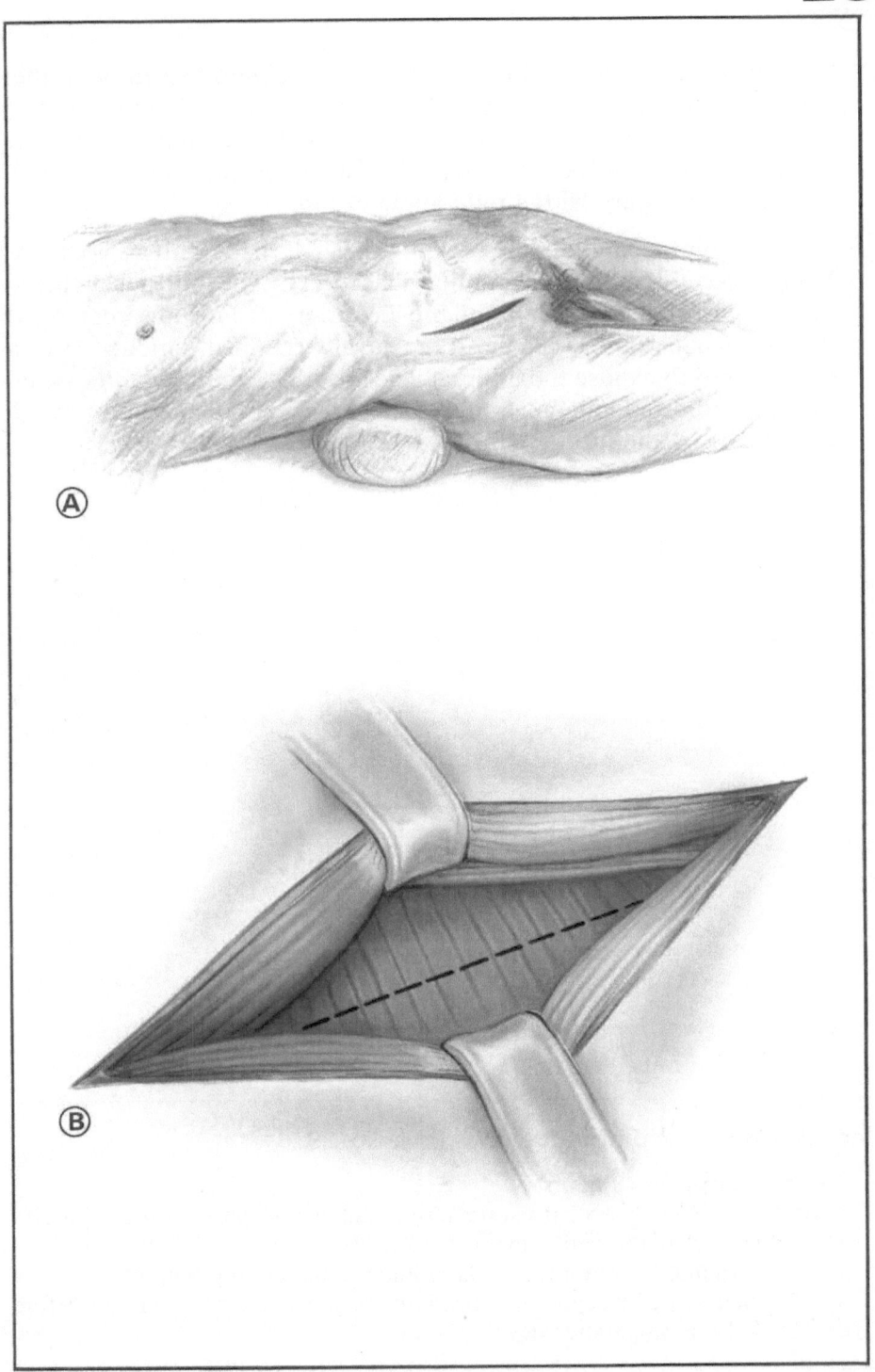

Ⓑ

Ⓒ After oblique cutting of the internal oblique abdominal muscle, the peritoneum is pushed in a medial direction and held aside with a retractor. At the top in the picture, a loop has been placed around the ureter and it is held to one side. In the picture, a loop is being placed on the common iliac artery with a right angle clamp.

Ⓓ After further preparation, the ureter is also held aside with a spatula. A loop is placed around the common iliac artery. After further preparation, a loop can be placed around the iliac artery (facing upwards). Now the external iliac artery can be atraumatically clamped. This access can also be used to expose the internal iliac artery and to ligate it in case of bleeding from an inoperable carcinoma of the rectum, in case of severe bleeding from the uterine artery.

Postoperative Recommendations from No. 29

- Redon drainage for 48 hours.
- Antibiotic shield with 3 x 2.0 g or 6 x 1.0 g Cefamandole, possibly other antibiotics (depending on the antibiogram) for 5 days.
- 3 x 5000 U depot heparin per day, later anticoagulation not required.
- Mobilization only after septic complications are under control, that is, not before the 3rd or 4th postoperative day.

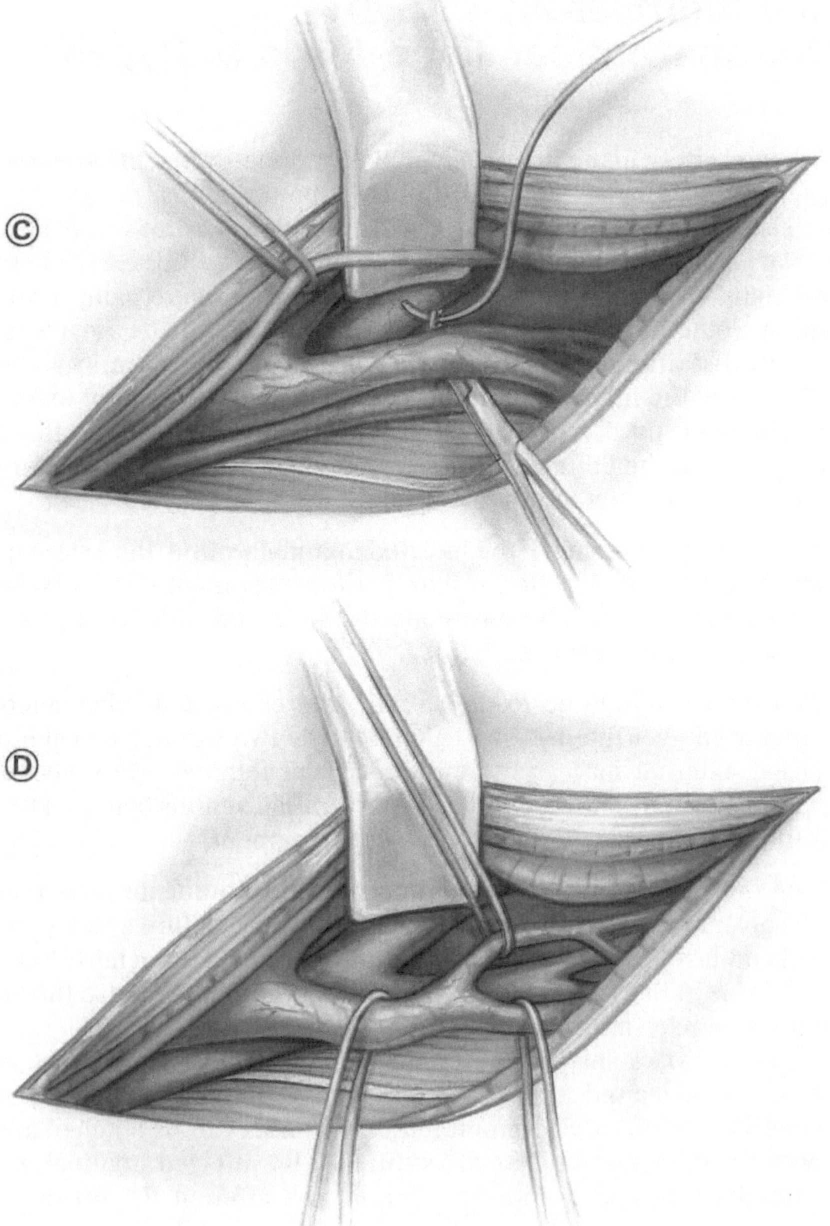
C
D

29

Spanning an Infected Vascular Wound in the Right Groin with an Extra-anatomical Iliaco-femoral Bypass

The femoral artery in the inguinal region is undoubtedly at the greatest risk with regard to vascular infection (infected lymph nodes, peripheral gangrene, skin contamination). Here, we will describe a possible way to proceed in case of an infected inguinal vascular wound. Diagnosis is easy. There are typical signs of infection with redness, swelling, pressure pain, fever and pulsation. Sometimes smaller prodromal hemorrhages to the outside reveal severe, profuse arterial bleeding. To be able to save the extremity and to be able to control the infection induced bleeding, the technique of extra-anatomical bypass is used. It can be performed not only laterally, as in this case, but also through the obturator foramen. We have collected satisfactory experiences with the method of lateral bypass.

Ⓐ After careful covering of the infected inguinal wound, the external iliac artery is exposed thorough an extraperitoneal point of access (28) and in the picture, it is already anastomosed side-to-end with the large saphenous vein taken from the left leg.

Ⓑ The bypass should be made laterally and conducted subcutaneously downward over the inguinal ligament. The two wounds reveal the exposed external iliac artery and superficial femoral artery above the adductor canal. They are linked by the grafted venous bypass. The broken lines indicate the infected vascular segment.

Ⓒ The superficial femoral artery is exposed after cutting the large femoral fascia and blunt partition of the adductor musculature and anastomosed end-to-side with the bypass. It should be noted that a fairly long section of vein has to be removed from the other leg, because the lateral rerouting uses more material.
When the extra-anatomical venous bypass has been grafted, the infected inguinal wound, after changing the covering, can be opened and the superficial and deep common femoral arteries can be stitched around with thick Vicryl® or Dexon® sutures. The infected inguinal wound should be equipped with an efferent and afferent Redon drainage, through which is can be washed with antibiotic solution.

Postoperative Reccomendations see p. 154.

Ⓐ

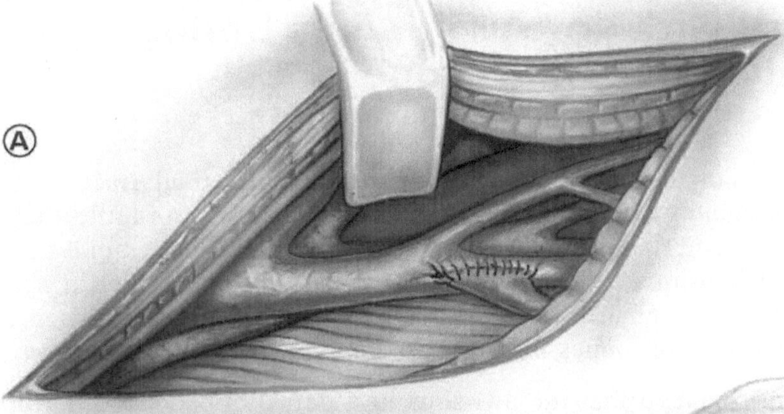

Ⓑ

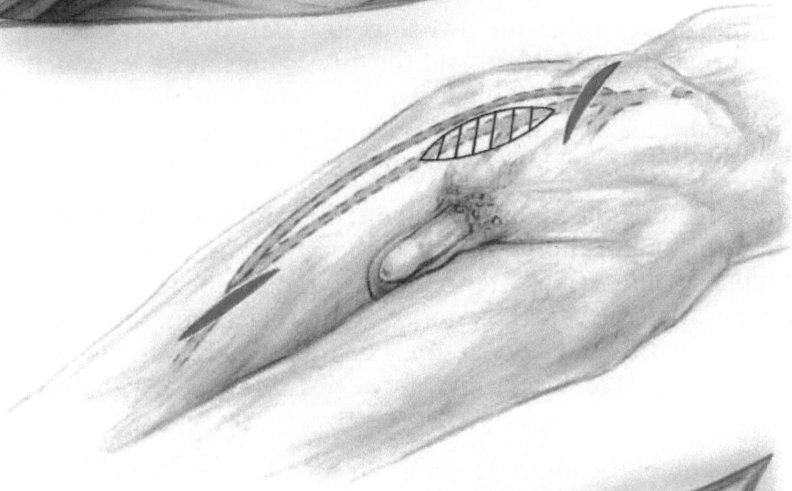

Ⓒ

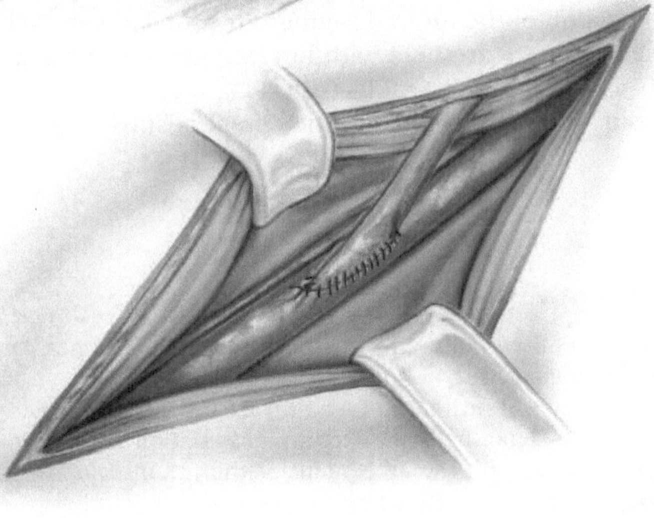

30

Injury of the Superficial Femoral/Popliteal Artery with an "Awl" While Boring Through the Thigh Bone

A common method of dealing with a pertrochanteric thigh fracture simply and with stability against loads is Ender's elastic nailing. As a rule, these are old patients and stabilization of the fracture must take place rapidly. After a small skin incision on the inner side of the distal end of the thigh, it is necessary to bore through the cortex. As a rule, this is readily accomplished, especially with the soft bones of aged persons.

Ⓐ It may happen that the awl slips in a dorsal direction during boring (eburnation of the bone, old fracture, clumsiness), in which case, the superficial femoral-popliteal artery or vein running at that point may be injured. This results in profuse bleeding, which cannot be pinpointed because of the adductor musculature that lies over it.

Ⓑ After cutting the adductor tendon, the popliteal artery can be palpated and the site of the injury can be located. Atraumatic clamps may be applied. Quite often, arteriosclerotic changes are found in this region (a site with predilection for arteriosclerotic occlusional disease) so that calcium deposits and stenoses may be found in the vascular wall. For this reason, direct measures may not be possible to deal with the site of injury and

Ⓒ resection of the injured segment must take place. The edges of the resected artery are held with holding threads-grafting of a piece of vein from the large saphenous vein is planned (see No. 19). In injuries of the vein, popliteal ligature of the vessel is sufficient.

Postoperative Measures

- Palpation of the pulse after the operation several times per day.
- Redon drainage for 48 hours.
- Antibiotic shield with 2 x 2.0 g or 4 x 1.0 g Cefamandole for 3 days.
- 3 x 5000 U depot heparin, later anticoagulation not required.
- Mobilization, with the agreement of the traumatologist on 2nd postoperative day.

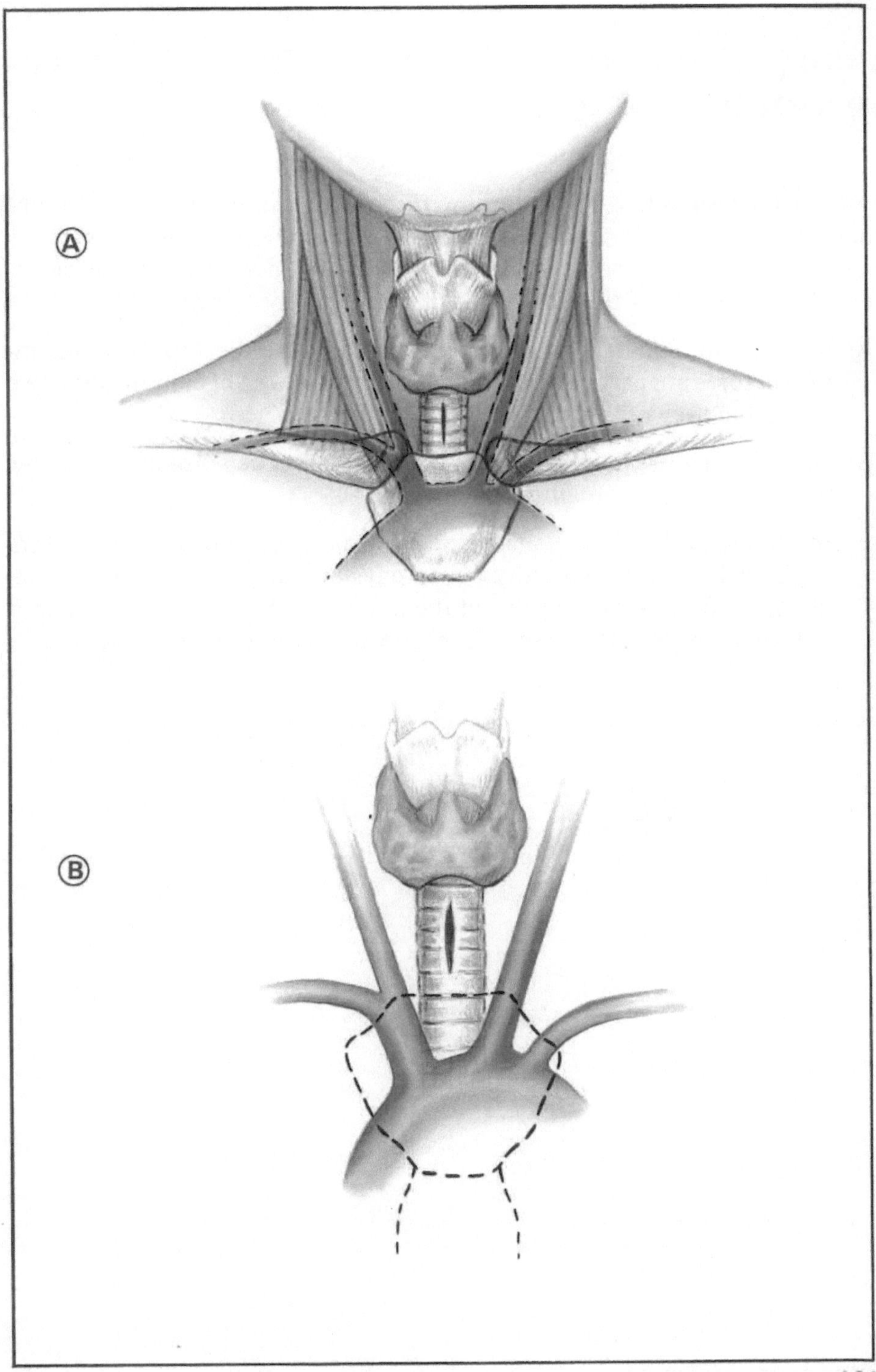
A
B

31

Injury of the Right Common Carotid Artery in Tracheotomy

We will not discuss here the indication for a tracheotomy – there is no doubt that there is such an indication in a large number of gravely ill patients who have to be intubated and ventilated over prolonged periods. Nor will we enter into the details of the technique of tracheotomy here.

Ⓐ Normal site. The incision for the tracheotomy is indicated. The anatomic structures are parted, allowing a tracheotomy free of complication (we prefer the "sewn-in" type of tracheotomy).

Ⓑ Normal depature points of the supra-aortic-branches-broken lines show the outlines of the manubrium sterni.

In a few cases (ca. 1–5%), there is severe arterial bleeding while performing a tracheotomy (sometimes even days or weeks later due to inflammatory softening of the walls of the large vessels of the neck, which is more common in the case of a tracheostoma that is not "sew in".

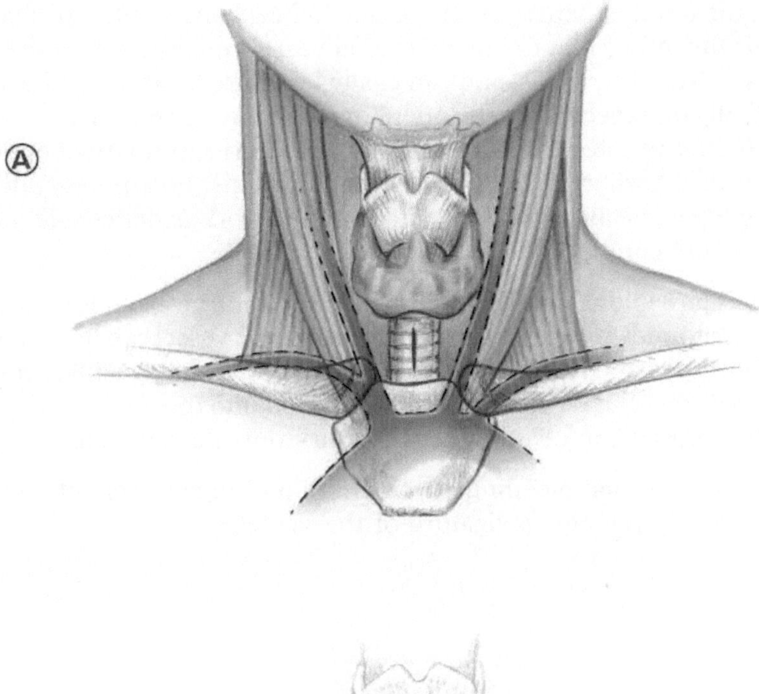
A
B

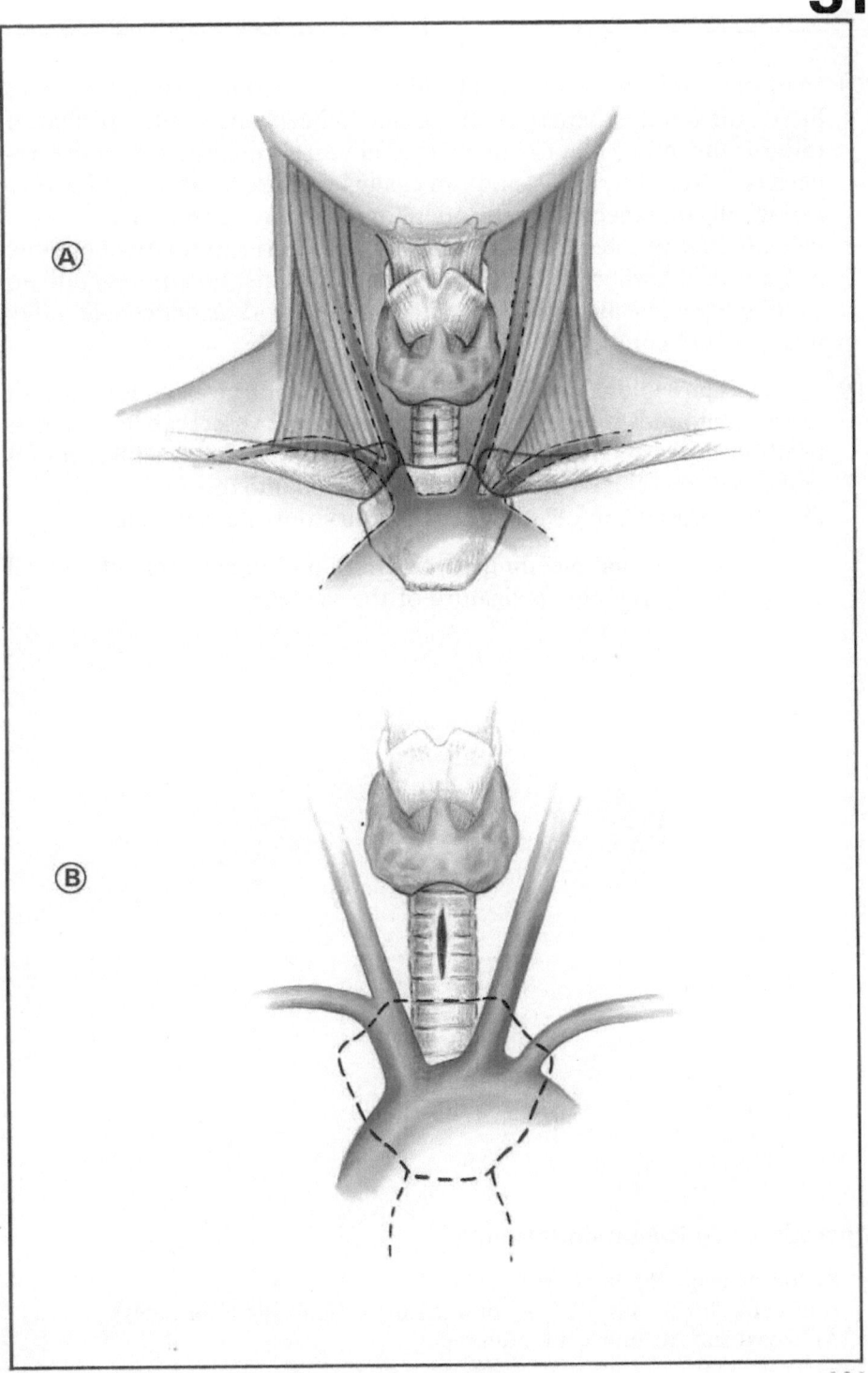

Ⓒ In most such cases of arterial bleeding, there is some anatomical peculiarity; the point of departure of the bracheocephalic trunk is displaced towards the left so that the main arterial vessel runs in front of the trachea (see No. 31 B, p. 161) and can easily be injured. Bleeding is severe and wholly unexpected for the operator (the more so since the anesthetists on duty in intensive care units have to perform the tracheotomy at the bedside, where there is no adequate lighting, no aspirator and no satisfactory assistance and the operator has to work under considerably disorganized conditions).

Ⓓ Once it is possible at least to install a good light and an aspirator, the particular anatomical situation can be identified, the vessel can be atraumatically clamped and the site of injury can be closed simply with monofilament sutures. Next, the skin should be sewn into the tracheostoma so that the sutured site of the vascular injury remains covered.

In case of erosional bleeding after a more prolonged tracheotomy, all that obviously remains is ligature of the vessel.

Postoperative Recomendations

- Redon drainage for 48 hours.
- Antibiotic shield with 2 x 2.0 g or 4 x 1.0 g Cefamandole for 3 days.
- Anticoagulant treatment not required.

Ⓒ

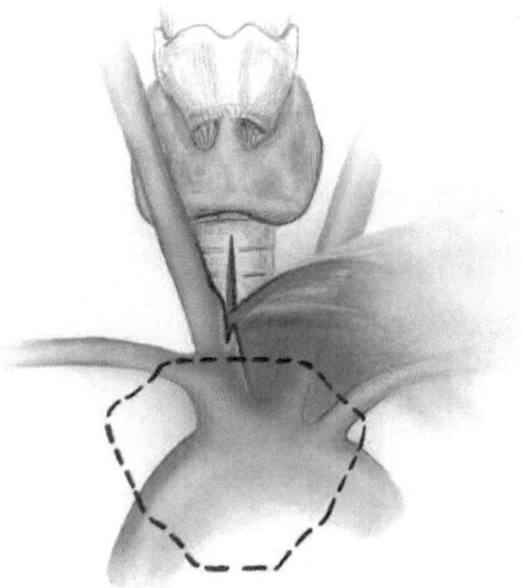

Ⓓ

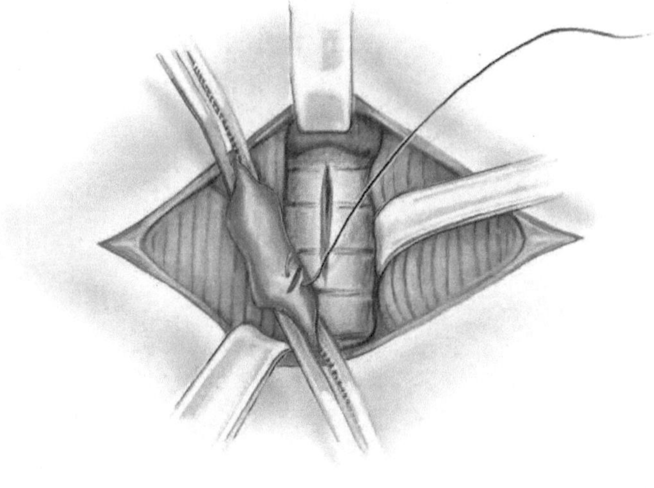

References

Bell, P. R. F., Tilney, N. L.: Vascular Surgery. (Internat. Med. Reviews.) Sevenoaks: Butterworth. 1984.

Bergan, J. J.: Arterial Surgery. Edinburgh: Churchill Livingstone. 1984.

Buri, P.: Traumatologie der Blutgefäße. Bern-Stuttgart-Wien: H. Huber. 1973.

Chang, J. B. (ed.): Vascular Surgery. (SP Medical and Scientific Books.) Jamaica, N. Y.: Spectrum. 1985.

Cooley, D. A., Wukasch, D. C.: Gefäßchirurgie, Technik und Indikation. (German version by Lick, R. F.) Stuttgart: Schattauer. 1980.

Heinrich, P.: Gefäßchirurgie, München-Berlin-Wien: Urban und Schwarzenberg. 1976.

Kappert, K.: Lehrbuch und Atlas der Angiologie, 10th ed. Bern-Stuttgart-Wien: H. Huber. 1981.

May, R.: Chirurgie der Bein- und Beckenvenen. Stuttgart: G. Thieme. 1974.

Moore, W. S.:Vascular Surgery: A Comprehensive Review. Orlando, Fla.: Grune & Stratton. 1983.

Pernkopf E.: Atlas der topographischen und angewandten Anatomie des Menschen, Vol. II. München-Berlin: Urban und Schwarzenberg. 1964.

Podlaha, H., Haaf, E.: Manual der peripheren Arterienoperationen. Stuttgart: F. Enke. 1974.

Vogt, B.: Gefäßverletzungen mit besonderer Berücksichtigung der peripheren Arterientraumatologie. Bern-Stuttgart-Wien: H. Huber. 1975.

Vollmar, J.: Rekonstruktive Chirurgie der Gefäße, 3rd ed. Stuttgart: G. Thieme. 1982.

Ward, A. S., Cormier, J. M.: Operative Techniques in Arterial Surgery. Baltimore, Md.: University Park Press. 1985.

Wylie, E. J., Stoney, R. J., Ehrenfeld, W. K.: Manual of Vascular Surgery, Vol. I. Berlin-Heidelberg-New York: Springer. 1980.